Case Presentations for the MRCS and AFRCS

Titles in the series

Case Presentations for the MRCS and AFRCS

Volume 1

Edited by

Philip Hornick BSc, MBBChir, FRCS
Lecturer, Department of Cardiothoracic Surgery,
Hammersmith Hospital, London

John Lumley MS, FRCS
Professor of Surgery, Professorial Surgical Unit,
St Bartholomew's Hospital, London

Pierce Grace MCh, FRCSI, FRCS
Professor of Surgical Science, University of Limerick,
Limerick

A member of the Hodder Headline Group
LONDON · NEW YORK · NEW DELHI

This edition first published in Great Britain in 1997 by Butterworth Heinemann.

This impression published by Arnold,
A member of the Hodder Headline Group,
338 Euston Road, London NW1 3BH

http://www.arnoldpublishers.com

Distributed in the USA by
Oxford University Press Inc.,
198 Madison Avenue, New York, NY10016
Oxford is a registered trademark of Oxford University Press

© 1997 Arnold

Whilst the advice and information in this book are believed to be true and accurate at the date of going to press, neither the authors nor the publisher can accept any legal responsibility or liability for any errors or omissions that may be made. In particular (but without limiting the generality of the preceding disclaimer) every effort has been made to check drug dosages; however, it is still possible that errors have been missed. Furthermore, dosage schedules are constantly being revised and new side-effects recognized. For these reasons the reader is strongly urged to consult the drug companies' printed instructions before administering any of the drugs recommended in this book.

British Library Cataloguing in Publication Data
A catalogue record for this book is available from the British Library

Library of Congress Cataloging-in-Publication Data
A catalog record for this book is available from the Library of Congress

ISBN 0 7506 3257 7

What do you think about this book? Or any other Arnold title?
Please send your comments to feedback.arnold@hodder.co.uk

Contents

Contributors

Reyad Al-Ghnaniem
King's College School of Medicine and Dentistry,
University of London, London

Peter Alton BSc, MB, BS, MRCP, DipRCPath
Lecturer in Haematology, St Georges Hospital, London

Peter Baird FRCS
Consultant Orthopaedic Surgeon, Charing Cross Hospital,
London

Irving S. Benjamin BSc, MD, FRCS
Professor of Surgery, King's College School of Medicine and
Dentistry, University of London, London

Patrick Broe MCh, FRCSI
Consultant Surgeon, Beaumont Hospital, Dublin, Ireland

Lesley Bromley BSc, MB, BS, FRCA, MHM
Senior Lecturer/Consultant Anaesthetist, Academic
Sub-department of Anaesthesia, University College
London Hospitals, The Middlesex Hospital, London

Paul Brookes BSc
Senior Biomedical Scientist, Department of Immunology,
Royal Postgraduate Medical School, Hammersmith
Hospital, London

W. Burgoyne BSc, FRCS
Senior House Officer in Plastic and Reconstructive Surgery,
Academic Department of Surgery, The Rayne Institute,
University College Hospitals NHS Trust, London

Robert Cocks MS, FRCS (Ed)
Consultant in Accident and Emergency, Hammersmith
Hospital, London

Claire Cousins FRCR
Consultant Radiologist, Hammersmith Hospital, London

Tom Creagh BSc, MCh, FRCSI
Consultant Urologist, Kingston Hospital, London

D.P. Dutka MRCP
Research Fellow and Honorary Senior Registrar,
Department of Medicine (Clinical Cardiology), Royal
Postgraduate Medical School, Hammersmith Hospital, London

Jonathan Forty MA, FRCS
Senior Lecturer in Cardiothoracic Surgery, Freeman Hospital,
Newcastle upon Tyne

Justin Geoghegan MCh, FRCSI
Senior Registrar in Surgery, Beaumont Hospital, Dublin,
Ireland

Michael J. Gough MB, ChB, ChM, FRCS
Consultant Vascular Surgeon, The General Infirmary at Leeds,
Leeds

Paul A. Harris BSc, MB, BS, FRCS
Senior House Officer in Surgical Training, Department of
Surgery, Charing Cross Hospital, London

Ciaran Healy MD, DCH, FRCSI, FRCS(Plast)
Senior Registrar in Plastic and Reconstructive Surgery,
Academic Department of Surgery, The Rayne Institute,
University College Hospitals NHS Trust, London

Charles Hinds FRCP, FRCA
Senior Lecturer and Consultant in Intensive Care,
Intensive Care Unit, St Bartholomew's Hospital, London

Claire Hornick
Transplant Coordinator, North Thames East, Charterhouse
Chambers, London

Philip Hornick BSc, MBBChir, FRCS
Lecturer, Department of Cardiothoracic Surgery,
Hammersmith Hospital, London

Sir Miles Irving MD, ChB, FRCS
Professor, University Department of Surgery, Hope Hospital,
Salford

Donald J. Jeffries BSc, MBBS, FRCPath
Professor, Department of Virology, The Medical College of
St Bartholomew's Hospital, University of London, London

E.M. Keily FRCSI, FRCS
Consultant Paediatric Surgeon, Great Ormond Street Hospital,
London

W. Kmiot MS, FRCS
Consultant Colorectal Surgeon, Hammersmith Hospital, London

Robert I. Lechler MBChB, PhD, FRCP
Head of Department and Honorary Consultant in Medicine,
Department of Immunology, Royal Postgraduate Medical
School, Hammersmith Hospital, London

John A. Lynn MS, FRCS
Consultant Endocrine Surgeon, Hammersmith Hospital, London

A.J. McCleary MA, BM, BCh, FRCS
Vascular Surgical Unit, The General Infirmary at Leeds, Leeds

J. MacFie MD, FRCS
Consultant Surgeon, Scarborough Hospital, Scarborough

Averil O. Mansfield ChM, FRCS
Professor, Academic Surgical Unit, St Mary's Hospital, London

Y. Mor MD
Senior Registrar, Department of Paediatric Urology,
Great Ormond Street Hospital, London

P.D.E. Mouriquand FRCS
Consultant Paediatric Urologist, Great Ormond Street Hospital,
London

P.M. Murchan FRCS
Department of Surgery, Scarborough Hospital, Scarborough

A. Ross Naylor MD, FRCS
Consultant Vascular Surgeon, Aberdeen Royal Infirmary,
Aberdeen

R. John Nicholls MChir, FRCS
St Mark's Hospital, Harrow, Middlesex

Michael O'Leary FRCA
Clinical Research Fellow in Intensive Care, St Bartholomew's
Hospital, London

Chandana Ratnatunga BSc, MS, FRCS(CTh)
Consultant Cardiac Surgeon, Department of Cardiothoracic
Surgery, Hammersmith Hospital, London

D.M. Richards MB, ChB, FRCS
Tutor in Surgery, Intestinal Failure Unit, Hope Hospital, Salford

Helena Scott BA, MB, BChir, FRCA
Registrar, Department of Anaesthesia, Hammersmith
Hospital, London

Humphrey Scott MS, FRCS
St Mark's Hospital, Harrow, Middlesex

David M. Scott-Coombes MS, FRCS
Consultant Endocrine Surgeon, King's College School of
Medicine and Dentistry, University of London, London

Ravinder Singh Nagra
Department of Surgery, Hammersmith Hospital, London

Dudley Sinnett FRCS
Consultant in Breast Surgery, Charing Cross Hospital, London

Alastair Skelly BSc, MBBS, FRCA
Consultant and Honorary Senior Lecturer, Department of
Anaesthesia, Hammersmith Hospital, London

Mark Smith BSc, MBBS, FRCA
Research Registrar, Department of Anaesthesia, Hammersmith
Hospital, London

Martin Smith FRCA
Consultant Neuroanaesthetist, Tavistock Surgical Intensive
Care Unit, The National Hospital for Neurology and
Neurosurgery, London

Peter Smith MRCP, FRCS
Consultant Cardiothoracic Surgeon, Hammersmith Hospital,
London

Christopher T.M. Speakman MD, FRCS
St Mark's Hospital, Harrow, Middlesex

John Spencer MS, FRCS
Consultant Surgeon, Hammersmith Hospital, London

Gerard Stansby MChir, FRCS
Senior Lecturer/Honorary Consultant Surgeon, Academic
Surgical Unit, St Mary's Hospital, London

Neil S. Tolley MD, FRCS, DLO
Consultant ENT/Head and Neck Surgeon, St Mary's and Ealing
NHS Trust, London

Thomas Noel Walsh MD, MCh, FRCSI
Department of Surgery, Beaumont Hospital, Dublin,
Ireland

Anthony N. Warrens BSc, BM, BCh, MRCP(UK)
MRC Clinician Scientist and Honorary Senior Registrar,
Renal Unit, Royal Postgraduate Medical School, Hammersmith
Hospital, London

J.D. Watson BSc, MBBS, FRCA
Consultant and Senior Lecturer, Anaesthesia and Intensive
Care Medicine, Homerton and St Bartholomew's Hospital,
London

Elizabeth Whitehead BSc, MB, FCAnaes
Consultant Anaesthetist, Ealing Hospital, Southall, Middlesex

R.C.N. Williamson MA, MD, MChir, FRCS
Director of Surgery, Royal Postgraduate Medical School,
Hammersmith Hospital, London

Preface

Postgraduate surgical training in the UK and Ireland has evolved to a new and more structured set point. The surgical colleges have introduced a number of new examinations – MRCS and AFRCS – to replace the old FRCS, which has become an intercollegiate exit examination. The new examinations specifically address surgical principles and practice and it is to the student approaching these written, oral and clinical assessments that this book is aimed. We chose the case history format as we consider it the most suitable and realistic medium for structured thought and clinically appropriate management.

When preparing for any examination, the candidate's continual wonder (and worry!) is 'what will they ask me?' and 'even if I know the answer, will it be enough?' To try and provide some insight into a prospective examiner's expectations we initially selected a broad range of topics from the syllabi of the new MRCS/AFRCS examinations. We then invited a large group of specialists, many of whom are examiners, to write case histories using a question-and-answer format at a level of knowledge that they would expect from a candidate for the MRCS/AFRCS examination. We asked that their histories be comprehensive, and to append a further reading list in order to provide the uninitiated reader with an overview, and an opportunity to read deeper into that particular condition. Their contributions, which emphasize basic surgical and scientific principles, form the basis of this book.

The mark of an expert is the ability to make one's own subject interesting and easily understood by everyone. This volume is a unique collection of surgical case histories written by experts for non-experts. The authors have done a magnificent job and we are delighted with the result. We hope that it will provide a flavour of the diversity of problems likely to be encountered during a lifetime in surgical practice, as well as indicating the 'height of the hurdles' which need to be jumped in order to pass the examinations. To the authors, on behalf of surgical examination candidates everywhere, we thank you.

P.H.
P.A.G.
J.S.P.L.

Acknowledgements

We would like to thank all the authors who have contributed so generously of their knowledge and time to this project. Without them this book would not exist.

We especially thank Mrs Vivienne Dignum, our literary co-ordinator, whose organization, enthusiasm and overall dedication made this book a reality.

Case 1 Aortic dissection

A 63-year-old man was admitted to casualty by his general practitioner with a suspected myocardial infarction. He described the pain as being of sudden onset and excruciating, and felt that it was radiating to between his shoulder blades. On examination he was tachycardic, cold and sweaty with a blood pressure of 190/130 mmHg and the casualty officer heard an early diastolic murmur. An ECG showed signs of left ventricular hypertrophy with no changes indicative of myocardial infarction. A posteroanterior chest radiograph showed widening of the mediastinum.

Questions

1. What are the likely diagnosis, pathophysiology and risk factors?
2. Briefly describe two systems of classification.
3. How should this be investigated further?
4. What is the significance of a diastolic murmur?
5. Describe the initial preoperative management.
6. What are the principles of surgical therapy and expected outcome?

Answers

1. Acute aortic dissection. The primary lesion is an intimal tear; blood enters the media which is cleaved proximally and distally into its inner two-thirds and outer third. The tear is the result of shear stress forces generated by the left ventricular ejection velocity and systemic arterial pressure. These forces cause fractional movement of aortic intima over media. Whilst intimal and medial abnormalities are important, medial degeneration may be the result of hypertension, eccentric jet of blood from a bicuspid aortic valve or ageing. Risk factors include hypertension, Marfan's syndrome, bicuspid aortic valve, pregnancy and surgery to the ascending aorta (as in aortic valve replacement).

2. The *DeBakey* classification: type I involves a proximal tear; both the ascending and descending aorta are involved. Type II involves a proximal tear with the dissection confined to the ascending aorta. Type III involves a tear beyond the origin of the subclavian artery, with the dissection confined to the descending aorta.

   The *Stamford* classification is newer and describes two forms: type A involves the ascending aorta regardless of whether the descending aorta is involved. Type B describes a dissection confined to the descending thoracic aorta. This system, whilst easier to remember, is not as useful as the DeBakey system for auditing the results of treatment on the basis of anatomical site of the tear.

3. For many years aortography was the only accurate diagnostic procedure for the evaluation of patients with suspected aortic dissection. More recently, computed tomography (CT), magnetic resonance imaging (MRI), transoesophageal echocardiography (TOE) and transthoracic echocardiography (TTE) have also been shown to be useful. Aortography is performed by retrograde catheter insertion through the femoral artery. The diagnosis of a dissection by aortography is made on the basis of direct or indirect signs. Direct signs include visualization of a double lumen or an intimal flap. The indirect signs include compression of the true aortic lumen by the false lumen, thickening of the aortic wall, abnormalities of branches and an abnormal position of the catheter in the aorta. An advantage of aortography is its ability to detect the presence of some of the complications of dissection, for example aortic regurgitation, and involvement of the proximal coronary arteries. In addition, some surgeons value a coronary angiogram if the patient previously had a history of angina.

   MRI CT scanning and echocardiography have demonstrated that aortography is not as accurate as once thought. Furthermore, disadvantages of aortography include the use of intravenous contrast, especially in the context of actual or impending acute tubular necrosis. It is invasive, it takes time to perform the study, and involves an angiography team.

   The sensitivities of MRI, CT and TOE are similar (over 90%); TTE has a lower sensitivity. The specificities of both TTE and TOE are lower than CT and MRI, mainly as a result of false-positive findings in the ascending aorta. MRI and CT are more sensitive than TTE but not TOE in detecting thrombus formation in the entire thoracic aorta. TOE and MRI are accurate at detecting an entry site and aortic regurgitation, which CT is not able to do.

For patients who are haemodynamically stable CT or MRI should be the investigation of choice. TOE should be reserved for patients who are haemodynamically unstable as it can be performed at the bedside.

4. The diastolic murmur may indicate aortic annulus involvement leading to severe incompetence of the aortic valve, in which case a valve replacement or a resuspension procedure will be required. The dissection may extend into or shear off aortic side branches. Rupture may occur of the false lumen through the thin outer media and adventitia. Death is due to rupture or ischaemia of viscera.

5. The patient should be monitored on a high-dependency or intensive care unit until transfer to a cardiothoracic unit can be made. Following insertion of a central line, arterial line and urinary catheter, blood should be drawn for baseline haematological and biochemical investigations. A cross-match of 10 units should be performed and consent for operation obtained. If the patient is in shock, fluid replacement using blood or colloid should be instituted using the central venous pressure for guidance (to a maximum of $10 \, cmH_2O$). A low urine output (less than 30 ml/h) may indicate hypoperfusion due to involvement of the renal artery or to fluid depletion. Assuming the latter, following adequate fluid replacement, a bolus (40–80 mg frusemide), should be followed by a dopamine infusion, at a renal dose (1–4 μg/kg per min). It is extremely important to lower the arterial pressure of a hypertensive patient and to lower the velocity of ventricular ejection. Sodium nitroprusside is an arterial vasodilator but increases the velocity of ventricular ejection as a result of the reflex tachycardia. It may however be combined with a beta-adrenergic blocker which will decrease the ejection velocity, and an end-point of a heart rate of 60 beats/min may be used. Intravenous beta-blockers should be used. An alternative is labetalol, which is an alpha- and beta-blocker which effectively lowers the arterial blood pressure as well as reducing the velocity of left ventricular ejection due to the negative chronotropic and inotropic effects.

6. Surgery is essential for all patients with type A dissections. The operation is performed through a median sternotomy

with use of cardiopulmonary bypass. Cannulation of the true lumen of the femoral artery gives unencumbered access to the distal ascending aorta or transverse arch for distal anastomosis. Venous return is achieved by using a right atrial cannula. This diverts all blood returning to the heart into the bypass machine and thence to the aortic cannula. After establishing systemic hypothermia the aorta is cross-clamped and the sight of the intimal tear is identified. The heart is protected from the deleterious effects of ischaemia by the administration of cardioplegia directly into the coronary ostia. The principles of surgical management for type A dissections are as follows:

(a) Aortic regurgitation must be eliminated by either resuspension or replacement of the aortic valve. If there is dissection around the valve annulus, the valve will need to be resuspended if it is normal, and replaced if it is abnormal (e.g. bicuspid, or accompanied by Marfan's syndrome).

(b) The false lumen should be obliterated at the proximal extent of the dissection, which is the most likely site of rupture.

(c) Intimal continuity should be re-established by either resecting or excluding the site of the intimal tear (the entry site) and interposing a vascular graft sewn proximally and distally to the full thickness of the aortic wall. In the majority of patients the false lumen will remain patent distally because of multiple re-entry sites. This is beneficial because organ perfusion through major vessels may depend on the false lumen flow.

(d) In those cases when the tear extends into the aortic arch, failure to resect it does not appear to affect outcome. Aortic arch replacement may be required if flow into the carotid or subclavian vessels has been compromised by the dissection, or if impending rupture of the arch is likely.

For type B dissections, conservative management should be instituted, as surgery confers no additional benefit in the absence of complications. Complications requiring operative intervention are bleeding, visceral ischaemia, uncontrollable hypertension, neurological deficits, persistent pain, arterial compromise, expansion or rupture.

Following operation for a type A dissection, the in-hospital mortality is approximately 70–90%, with a 10-year survival rate of 30–40%. In the case of type B dissections in the absence of complications, operation does not appear to confer any survival benefit over and above medical therapy alone.

Further reading

Crawford ES. (1990) The diagnosis and management of aortic dissection. *Journal of the American Medical Association* **264**: 2537–2541

Philip Hornick
Peter Smith

Case 2 Renal failure

A 60-year-old woman, found to have a cholangiocarcinoma, underwent a partial hepatectomy. Three days later she became pyrexial and was treated with cefuroxime and gentamicin, following which the fever settled. Two days after this, by which time she was profoundly icteric, it was noted that her previously normal serum creatinine had risen to 184 μmol/l. The next day it had climbed further to 265 μmol/l and her urine output had begun to decrease.

Questions

1. What is the differential diagnosis of this woman's renal impairment?
2. What investigations might help you confirm the diagnosis?
3. For each differential diagnosis, what is the likely renal prognosis?

Answers

1. It is not possible to be certain why this woman's renal function deteriorated but this case does offer a useful opportunity to review the approach to renal failure in the postoperative patient. It is well known that impaired renal function may be of prerenal, renal or postrenal aetiology; in reality, when considering a differential diagnosis, it is often easiest to review them in the order: postrenal, prerenal and renal causes.

   (a) *Postrenal causes:* For the creatinine to rise in this fashion, both kidneys would have to be affected, since an unobstructed system will usually compensate for an obstructed contralateral kidney. This usually indicates a lesion at the level of the bladder or its outflow tract. It should be noted that an undiagnosed single kidney is quite common (one study reports a prevalence of 0.3%), in which case obstruction above the bladder could cause her creatinine to rise. However, there is no reason to suspect acute obstruction in this woman.

(b) *Prerenal causes:* Since there is no reported hypotension or blood loss, one may assume that none occurred, although in the postoperative patient this is common and must be looked for, particularly in the records of blood pressure during the anaesthetic and in the recovery room. Beware the 'normal' blood pressure in an elderly person with a history of hypertension. A pressure of 120/70 mmHg represents hypotension for someone used to preoperative values of 165/95 mmHg!

Patients who develop sepsis are at increased risk of developing acute tubular necrosis (ATN), and this may have contributed in this patient. However, her major risk factor for prerenal renal failure is her hepatic dysfunction. For reasons that are still incompletely understood, renal blood flow and glomerular filtration rate are severely impaired in liver failure. The kidneys respond to this in the same way as they might to a haemorrhage – by conserving salt and water. The patient may become uraemic and oliguric as a result, although the kidneys are structurally unimpaired. Indeed, if hepatic function improves, the renal function will return to normal. This is known as the hepatorenal syndrome. It is essentially a form of functional prerenal uraemia.

(c) *Intrinsic renal causes:* ATN is the end-result of prolonged hypotension, and represents the end-point of prerenal renal failure. ATN differs from prerenal uraemia in that the renal dysfunction is now not immediately reversible. This reversibility can only be assessed by removing the underlying cause and ensuring normal renal blood flow. When established ATN does occur, a unifying feature is the failure of the kidney to concentrate solute, resulting in high sodium and low urea concentrations in the urine. This may be in the context of either low urine output (oliguria) or not. Indeed, some patients often pass large volumes of urine when in ATN. It is also common for patients who have been oliguric subsequently to develop polyuria. With a normal glomerular filtration rate of 100 ml/min, renal blood flow is 144 l/24 h; if that is reduced to 3% of normal, in the absence of any concentrating ability, the patient will still pass 4.32 l of urine.

There are two potential causes for ATN in this case: sepsis (as mentioned above) and gentamicin therapy. Gentamicin is nephrotoxic and renally excreted. There are no blood levels given to confirm whether or not toxic levels were reached in this patient. However, gentamicin usually causes patients to develop polyuric ATN, without ever passing through an oliguric phase – this patient was becoming oliguric, making this diagnosis less likely.

The final possibility to be considered is that one of the drugs administered has precipitated an acute tubulo-interstitial nephritis (often known simply as acute interstitial nephritis, AIN). Both cefuroxime and gentamicin can do this, and it is likely that she will have received other agents.

   (d) *Differential diagnosis*
      (i)   Hepatorenal syndrome.
      (ii) Prerenal uraemia due to sepsis.
      (iii) ATN due to sepsis.
      (iv) ATN due to gentamicin.
      (v) AIN due to cefuroxime, gentamicin or another unmentioned drug.

2. If this is prerenal uraemia, such as the hepatorenal syndrome or due to dehydration, the kidneys' tubules will be retaining sodium and water. Thus the urinary concentration of sodium will be low while the urea concentration and osmolality will be high. These tests are done on a 'spot' urine: it is not necessary to take a 24-h collection such as is used for a formal measurement of creatinine clearance. Table 2.1 shows the ranges within which these data will be helpful. Between these ranges, they are difficult to interpret.

Table 2.1

	Oliguric acute renal failure	Prerenal uraemia
Urinary sodium concentration (U_{Na}; mmol/l)	>40	<20
Urinary urea concentration (mmol/l)	<150	>150
Urinary osmolality (mosmol/kg H_2O)	<350	>500
Urine/plasma osmolality	<1.1	>1.5
Urinary (U_{Cr}) to plasma (P_{Cr}) creatinine ratio	<20	>40
Renal failure index = $U_{Na}/(U_{Cr}/P_{Cr})$	>1	<1

Another way in which useful information might be gathered from examination of the urine is by dipstick analysis and microscopy. The leakage of protein in the absence of blood is highly suggestive of intrinsic renal disease.

Haematuria is less useful at localizing a problem as many lesions in the urinary tract may bleed. However, microscopy might identify the presence of pathological casts, again suggestive of a problem within the kidneys.

Urine microscopy might be a valuable tool in diagnosing AIN. Being associated with active inflammation, white cells and white cell casts may be seen on urine microscopy in AIN. Sometimes eosinophils may be seen, underlining the allergic basis of this lesion. The absence of these findings does not exclude the diagnosis of AIN. These findings would not be present in ATN or prerenal uraemia.

If the diagnosis of AIN is considered to be likely, the only way to confirm the diagnosis with certainty would be to perform a percutaneous renal biopsy. AIN is rather low on the list of differential diagnoses in this case and renal biopsy is not indicated. The diagnosis of ATN can also be confirmed on biopsy, but it is usually sufficient initially to base this diagnosis on the evolution of the clinical picture and its response to intervention.

3. In the hepatorenal syndrome, the prognosis for the return of renal function depends on the prognosis of the liver disease: if the jaundice is reversed, the kidneys will return to normal function. Indeed, a kidney from an individual with the hepatorenal syndrome will function normally if transplanted into an otherwise normal recipient!

In prerenal uraemia, if ATN has not yet become established, the metabolic problem will reverse if the precipitant is removed, for example following an infusion of colloid. But even in established ATN, in an individual with normal premorbid renal function, the vast majority will return to normal or near-normal renal function within a period of days to weeks.

Finally, in AIN the prognosis is less certain. Most patients, even those requiring dialysis, do recover renal function if the precipitating agent is withdrawn, although this may be slow (up to a year) and incomplete.

Further reading

Cronin RE. (1985) The patient with acute azotemia. In: Schrier RW (ed.) *Manual of Nephrology*, pp. 133–146. Little, Brown, Boston

10

Epstein M. (1993) Hepatorenal syndrome. In: Lazarus JM and Brenner BM (eds) *Acute Renal Failure*, 3rd edn, pp. 527–552. Churchill Livingstone, New York

López-Novoa JM and Diez J. (1992) Acute renal failure in liver disease: clinical, diagnostic, and therapeutic aspects. In: Cameron JS, Davison AM and Grunfield JP (eds) *Oxford Textbook of Clinical Nephrology*, vol. 2, pp. 1098–1109. Oxford Medical Publications, Oxford

Anthony N. Warrens

Case 3 Scoring on the intensive care unit

A 69-year-old man was admitted to the intensive care unit
(ICU) from the operating theatres following emergency surgery for faecal peritonitis due to a perforated sigmoid diverticulum. He had a past history of severe rheumatoid arthritis
for which he had been on long-term treatment with prednisolone and non-steroidal anti-inflammatory agents. On admission
to the ICU his observations and blood results revealed the
following:

Temperature: 35.8°C   Pulse: 106 beats/min regular
BP 110/60 mmHg   Respirations: 12 breaths/min
                             (ventilated)
Glasgow Coma Score: not assessable in view of sedation
Urine output last 24 h: unknown
Blood count: Hb 10.0 g/dl   WBC 5.0 × 10^9/l
Arterial blood gases on 40% oxygen: pH 7.31, Pao_2 17 kPa,
    $Paco_2$ 4.5 kPa
Biochemistry: Na^+ 122 mmol/l K^+ 4.2 mmol/l
                creatinine 210 mmol/l

He had a right internal jugular catheter for measurement of
central venous pressure and to permit infusion of low-dose
dopamine to maintain urine output. He also had an intra-
arterial cannula and urinary catheter *in situ*. He was treated
with broad-spectrum antibiotics, steroid replacement and
intravenous fluids.

Four hours later his blood pressure had fallen to 75/35 mmHg
despite volume replacement. He was oliguric. The heart rate
had increased to 120 beats/min, temperature to 38.9°C and
blood gases revealed pH 7.29, Pao_2 8.0 kPa on 60% oxygen and
$Paco_2$ 4.2 kPa. A pulmonary artery (Swan–Ganz) catheter was
inserted and he was found to be vasodilated with a high cardiac output, characteristic of septic shock. Following introduction of a noradrenaline infusion his blood pressure
improved and he again began to pass urine.

12

Questions

1. How might this patient's severity of illness be quantified on admission? Which scoring system would you choose to make this assessment, and why?
2. How can the APACHE scoring systems be used to estimate this patient's risk of death?
3. Late on the first day of ICU stay the surgeon responsible for the patient considers that his chances of survival are negligible, and suggests that it might be appropriate to withdraw treatment. Can this decision be made on the basis of a severity of illness score for this patient?
4. What criticisms can be levelled at prognostic scoring systems?
5. You are responsible for a research project testing a new intervention in septic, critically ill patients. How would you utilize scoring in the design of your project? Which scoring system would you choose?

Answers

1. Clinicians have always used their medical knowledge, combined with past experience, to make predictions of likely patient outcome, but it is well recognized that the accuracy and utility of such subjective estimates are limited, in particular because human predictions are heavily influenced by recent experience. Frequently even experienced clinicians will differ when assessing prognosis and in this case, for example, the referring surgeon assessed the patient's chances as slim, whilst the intensive care staff were rather more optimistic.

   In recent years a variety of objective scoring systems have been developed in an attempt to estimate prognosis more accurately by using objective criteria derived from large patient databases. These scoring systems are generally based on an assessment of the severity of the patient's illness. Initially such assessments were obtained, for example, by quantifying the extent of injury in burns, the degree of neurological dysfunction following head injury (Glasgow Coma Score; GCS) and the severity of acute pancreatitis (Ranson Score). Unfortunately, because patients in intensive care are a heterogeneous population, usually with multi-system involvement, such disease-specific assessments have limited applicability. The severity of illness can be assessed by scoring the extent of therapeutic intervention required (Therapeutic Intervention Scoring System; TISS) but because physicians may differ in their therapeutic approach to critically ill patients, and unit policies vary from one hospital to another, such systems are not useful for between-unit comparisons.

It has been clearly demonstrated that during critical illness the degree of derangement of physiological variables from normal is closely related to subsequent hospital mortality, and that this applies across a wide range of medical and surgical conditions. The important variables have been identified either by an 'expert panel' and subsequently tested in a previously accumulated database, or by regression analysis of the characteristics of survivors and non-survivors in such a database. In addition to the acute physiological derangement, outcome is influenced by the patient's pre-existing physiological reserve. Age and certain chronic diseases, not necessarily related to the disease leading to ICU admission, are independent predictors of outcome from acute illness, and evidence suggests that where old age and a chronic condition occur together, their influence on outcome is additive. Chronic diseases are very common in the ICU population, but it appears that only those diseases which reduce an individual's immune response (such as the long-term steroid therapy administered to the patient described above) and severe organ system insufficiency significantly increase the risk of death. The nature of the acute illness also has important implications for outcome. Diabetic ketoacidosis, for example, induces a profound disturbance of physiology, yet is eminently treatable and has a low mortality in western countries, whereas coma due to a massive intracerebral haemorrhage may result in little physiological disturbance but has a high mortality. For a given degree of physiological derangement septic shock is also associated with a higher than average mortality. If an intensive care scoring system is to be useful in clinical practice it must incorporate only those variables which are readily available to physicians in all units, which can be measured objectively and which are obtainable at or close to the time of ICU admission.

Scoring systems based on the extent of the acute physiological derangement include the Acute Physiology, Age and Chronic Health Evaluation (APACHE) score, the Simplified Acute Physiology Score (SAPS) and the Mortality Prediction Model (MPM). The APACHE prognostic scoring system was described in 1981 by Knaus and colleagues. The score was refined in 1985 as APACHE II and further refined in 1989 as APACHE III. APACHE allocates points to a series of physiological variables according to the degree to which they differ from normal to produce an acute physiology score. In the original APACHE score 34 variables were scored; these were reduced to 12 in 1985 and expanded slightly to 17 in 1989. To the acute physiology score are added additional points for age and chronic health problems. APACHE II also takes account of whether a patient was an elective or an emergency surgical admission or a non-surgical admission, and the patient is allocated to one of 34 admission diagnoses. APACHE III has been expanded to consider the source of patient (accident and emergency, ward, operating theatre, other ICU) and 78 principal diagnoses. APACHE II scores range from 0 to 59 and APACHE III from 0 to 299. Higher scores indicate greater derangement from normal, although APACHE II scores of greater than 40 are very unusual.

The accuracy of APACHE II has been extensively validated throughout the world. Although the refined APACHE III system appears to have some small advantages in predictive accuracy over its predecessor, the software is not readily available, there is much greater worldwide experience with the use of APACHE II, and it is probably the most appropriate scoring system for use in our patient.

2. The prognosis for an individual patient can be estimated by weighting the APACHE II score according to the patient's diagnostic category and, in APACHE III, the source of the patient. The coefficients used have been derived from large patient databases. The APACHE III predictive estimates, for example, are based on a database of 17 440 patients, the score being converted to a probability of hospital mortality using individual logistic regression equations for each of the diagnoses and patient origins. It is important to note, however, that the APACHE II methodology cannot be applied at times other than the first 24 h of intensive care, and best accuracy is obtained when the worst acute physiology score during the first 24 h is used in the calculation.

In contrast, APACHE III risks of death can be calculated daily. For our patient, the predicted risk of death based on the worst APACHE II score in the first 24 h of admission was 34%.

3. Although APACHE and other severity scoring systems can be used to provide an estimate of risk of hospital death for individual patients, they do not predict outcome with certainty, and consequently should not be used in isolation as a basis for limiting or discontinuing treatment. Used as an aid to clinical judgement, however, outcome predictions may be of use, in that they take into account past experiences in an unbiased manner (in contrast to human decisions where recent experience has a disproportionate influence), they are based on reproducible data, and the database supporting the risk assessment is substantially larger than any one clinician's experience.

The Riyadh Intensive Care Program is a scoring system which is designed to produce a prediction of death for individual patients on a daily basis. The prediction is derived from a computerized trend analysis of a daily organ failure score (itself derived from the APACHE II score weighted according to the number and duration of organ failures); both the absolute score and daily rate of change are considered. Unfortunately, this system has not been shown to have good predictive accuracy when tested in different patient populations.

4. Prognostic scoring systems have been extensively criticized, especially when used to predict outcome in individual patients. Many are concerned that extrapolation of group statistics to individual outcome prediction is intrinsically unsound since, for example, additional information likely to influence outcome will be available to the clinician but not to the model. In practice, however, this criticism seems to be offset by the greater objectivity of scoring systems. Clearly it is important that the individual patient or patient population in question is comparable to the population from which the original database was derived, i.e. there is no selection bias. This could be a problem when scoring systems are applied across national boundaries, and there has been some concern that the patient databases for the APACHE scores originate in the USA and may not apply to other countries. Studies from New Zealand, the UK and Ireland, however, have suggested that in general this is not the case.

Clearly the validity of a prediction is crucially dependent on accurate data collection. This requires motivated, well-informed staff and simple forms or computer entry which can be completed rapidly. Ideally, data collection should fall to one or two specified individuals on a unit who understand in detail the principles underlying the scoring system. Even with special training, however, clinically important errors in acute physiology scores have been detected in up to 18% of cases.

The timing of resuscitation, the quality of the treatment given and the patient's response can all influence the accuracy of outcome prediction. First, all patients may not have received equally effective therapies. Second, the time course of a patient's response is variable, so it is unclear how soon after institution of therapy a prognostic score is most valid. APACHE II, for example, was found to underestimate the mortality of patients admitted to the ICU from other critical care areas within the hospital, perhaps because such patients have often deteriorated despite receiving appropriate treatment. Conversely, a seriously ill patient who has been effectively resuscitated on the ward may accrue a relatively low acute physiology score when scored after admission to intensive care. This factor is known as lead-time bias. The patient described in the case history, for example, had been partially resuscitated in the operating theatre, so his admission score may not have accurately reflected the severity of his illness. He deteriorated during the first 24 h of ICU admission, so a 'worst score in first 24 h' would probably be more accurate than an admission score. In this case the admission score was 18, whereas the worst score in 24 h was 24. It is now recommended, therefore, that 'worst in 24 h' scores should be used routinely. APACHE III incorporates a small adjustment which is designed to compensate for lead-time bias by taking into account the source of admission; patients admitted from other critical care areas, for example, are scored more heavily.

As already mentioned, the APACHE II methodology only applies during the first 24 h of ICU admission, and cannot be used to provide prognostic estimates at other times during the ICU stay. APACHE III, however, is designed to permit daily scoring and calculation of risk of death.

5. The intensive care population is heterogeneous and although many common pathways to organ dysfunction and even death are now recognized, especially in sepsis, the underlying pathologies and acute illness severity vary con-

17

siderably between individual patients, even within super-
ficially clear-cut diagnostic groups such as adult respiratory
distress syndrome and septic shock. Severity of illness
scoring using, for example, APACHE is a useful tool for
clinical research as it provides an objective measure of
equivalent illness severity between control and treatment
groups. Scoring is usually performed after randomization,
but patients may be scored before randomization in order to
stratify them according to illness severity, thereby ensuring
that risks are evenly distributed between groups. The power
of such comparisons can be enhanced by comparing
observed versus expected mortality rates in the two groups.
The expected mortality rate is estimated by dividing the
sum of the predicted risks of death for all patients by the total
number of patients, and the observed mortality rate is calculated by dividing the sum of actual deaths by the total
number of patients. The standardized mortality ratio (SMR)
can then be calculated by relating the observed to expected
rates of death. A SMR of greater than 1 suggests that fewer of
your patients are surviving than would be expected for the
severity of illness, whereas a SMR of less than 1 suggests that
a greater proportion than expected are surviving.

References and further reading

Boyd CR, Tolson MA and Copes WS. (1987) Evaluating trauma care: the TRISS
method. *Journal of Trauma* **27:** 370–378
Cullen DJ, Civetta JM, Briggs BA and Ferrera LC. (1974) Therapeutic intervention scoring system: a method for quantitative comparison of patient care.
Critical Care Medicine **2:** 57–60
Keene AR and Cullen DJ. (1993) Therapeutic intervention scoring system:
update 1993. *Critical Care Medicine* **11:** 1–3
Knaus WA, Draper EA, Wagner DP and Zimmerman JE. (1985) APACHE II: a
severity of disease classification system. *Critical Care Medicine* **13:** 818–829
Knaus WA, Wagner DP, Draper EA *et al.* (1991) The APACHE III prognostic
system: risk prediction of hospital mortality for critically ill hospitalised
adults. *Chest* **100:** 1619–1636
Knaus WA, Zimmerman JE, Wagner DP *et al.* (1981) APACHE – acute physiol-
ogy and chronic health evaluation: a physiologically based classification
system. *Critical Care Medicine* **9:** 591–597
Le Gall J. (1995) Severity scoring in the critically ill patient. In: Bone RC and
Vincent JL (eds) *Current Opinion in Critical Care*, vol. 1. Current Science,
Philadelphia, PA
Schuster DP and Kollef MH (eds) (1994) *Predicting Intensive Care Unit Outcome.*
Critical Care Clinics, January 1994. WB Saunders, Philadelphia, PA

Michael O'Leary and Charles Hinds

Case 4   Management of diabetes

A 60-year-old obese diabetic man presents for elective inguinal hernia repair. His diabetic control consists of careful diet and oral hypoglycaemic agents, namely glibenclamide 5 mg once daily and metformin 500 mg twice daily.

Questions

1. What features of the patient's medical history may be consequent upon his diabetes?
2. How would you determine the adequacy of the patient's preoperative diabetic control?
3. What adverse side-effects may occur as a result of the patient's diabetic therapy?
4. Describe the main differences between insulin-dependent (IDDM) and non-insulin-dependent (NIDDM) diabetics.
5. Discuss the pre- and postoperative management of the patient's non-insulin-dependent diabetes.

Answers

1. The complications of diabetics are a major cause of morbidity and mortality and may exert a significant influence on patient management and outcome. Atherosclerotic disease is common and in NIDDM accounts for 50% of the mortality. The main systems affected are:
   (a) *Cardiovascular:* Seek symptoms and signs of hypertension, ischaemic heart disease, peripheral and cerebral vascular disease.
   (b) *Renal:* Renal impairment may be present and can ultimately lead to renal failure.
   (c) *Nervous system:* Peripheral and autonomic neuropathies.
   (d) *Eyes:* Proliferative retinopathy and blindness.
2. The ideal result of diabetic therapy is the restoration of normal glucose tolerance. In order to assess glycaemic control, measurements of blood glucose concentrations are necessary. The levels of blood glucose that should be aimed for are shown in Table 4.1.

Table 4.1

Sample	Glucose
Blood	
Fasting	5.0 mmol/l
2 h postprandial	6.0 mmol/l
Preprandial	6.0 mmol/l
Urine	Negative

The patient scheduled for inguinal hernia repair should have a urine test and random blood glucose before surgery. If the blood glucose concentration is greater than 12 mmol/l, then the diabetic control is considered to be poor and the patient should be treated pre- and postoperatively as though he were insulin-dependent (see Volume 2, Case 4).

A useful guide to longer-term (2–6 weeks) control is the measurement of glycosylated haemoglobin (HbA_1C) which should be less than 10%. If it is greater than 10%, a longer period of stabilization of 48 h or more may be justified.

3. Hypoglycaemia is the most commonly observed adverse side-effect in the fasted patient awaiting surgery and can occur even when the morning dose of oral hypoglycaemic has been omitted. It is more readily observed in patients taking long-acting drugs such as chlorpropramide who have not previously been changed to a short-acting agent such as gliclazide.

   Lactic acidosis is a dangerous but uncommon complication of treatment with metformin. It should be suspected in patients who present with metabolic acidosis associated with a high anion gap, in the absence of severe ketoacidosis. It is usually prevented by avoidance of metformin treatment in patients with renal impairment, cardiac failure, hepatic dysfunction, peripheral vascular disease and chronic alcohol abuse, and by dosage reduction in patients taking H_2-receptor antagonists.

4. There are significant differences between IDDM diabetics (type I) and NIDDM diabetics (type II). The NIDDM patients are often older and prone to obesity. They are more likely to develop hyperosmolar coma than ketoacidosis. Their disease is characterized by a reduction in the number or function of insulin receptors. Amyloid deposition near the beta-cell membrane in NIDDM patients may be responsible for

defective insulin secretion and the insulin resistance seen in this disease.

IDDM diabetics tend to be younger (<35 years) and are more likely to develop ketoacidosis. In these cases beta-cell damage, probably secondary to viral injury or autoimmune mechanisms, results in failure of insulin secretion.

The incidence of long-term complications appears to differ in the two groups, possibly being related to the duration of the disease. There is a greater incidence of nephropathy and end-stage renal failure in IDDM, although microalbuminuria may be in existence at the time of the diagnosis of NIDDM and this predicts future cardiovascular and renal problems.

5. In a well-controlled diabetic taking only short- or medium-acting sulphonylureas, omission of the oral hypoglycaemic agent on the morning of elective minor surgery will usually suffice. In the case of long-acting sulphonylureas, e.g. chlorpropamide and the biguanide metformin, most texts recommend, wherever possible, their discontinuation 24–48 h preoperatively in order to minimize the risk of hypoglycaemia and lactic acidosis respectively. In these circumstances diabetic control should be retained with a short-acting sulphonylurea agent.

Close bedside monitoring of blood glucose levels using stick tests and, where available, reflectance meters is mandatory throughout the pre- and perioperative periods. It is sensible to ensure that the patient undergoes surgery as early as possible on a morning list, thus limiting the duration of fasting. Well-controlled diabetics on oral hypoglycaemic agents will not require any additional treatment unless major surgery is planned, or if it is expected that the patient will not be able to eat for more than 24 h postoperatively. Under these circumstances, glucose and insulin infusions should be set up and the patient treated as though he or she is an IDDM diabetic (see Volume 2, Case 4).

During surgery infusions which may induce hyperglycaemia, e.g. 5% glucose, are best avoided. Hartman's solution is also not recommended because of its lactate content. Postoperatively, blood glucose levels should continue to be monitored at the bedside. Oral hypoglycaemic agents may be reintroduced as soon as the patient has started eating.

Further reading

Milaskiewicz RH and Hall GM. (1992) Diabetes and anaesthesia: the past decade. *British Journal of Anaesthesia* **68:** 198–206

Elizabeth Whitehead

Case 5 Trauma and the ATLS system of care

A 75-year-old woman is involved in a road traffic accident in which she is struck by a bus whilst crossing the street. She is thrown against a concrete post by the force of the impact. At the scene she remains conscious and alert, complaining of pain in her right arm, which is clearly angulated and deformed. A dressing is applied to a large scalp wound and her head and neck are immobilized by the attending ambulance crew. An intravenous infusion is established in the left arm and an infusion of Ringer's lactate solution commenced. Supplemental oxygen is administered to the patient's face and she is rapidly transported to hospital.

On arrival at the accident and emergency department she is rapidly assessed by the trauma team. She is awake and alert but has a small amount of blood in her mouth from broken teeth. Her remaining dentures are removed. She is able to expectorate easily and with a pulse oximeter her Sao_2 is 100%. Her heart rate is 60 beats/min, with an impalpable radial pulse on her right arm and poorly palpable femoral pulses. The intravenous line is seen to have tissued. She is unable to move her legs when asked to do so and has no feeling in the lower half of her body. Her scalp wound is the only obvious source of overt blood loss and examination of her back when log-rolled reveals no other wound or abnormality.

Her family arrive in a highly agitated state and explain that the patient was previously in robust health save for requiring beta-blockade therapy for pre-existing hypertension. They confirm events from the scene of the accident.

Questions

1. Describe the initial resuscitative management of this lady.
2. Why might she have hypotension and bradycardia?
3. What X-rays should be undertaken to assist management?
4. Outline the principles of initial care for a paraplegic patient.
5. What scoring systems do you know which will describe this lady's injuries and help suggest her likelihood of survival?

Answers

1. This woman has suffered multiple trauma. She has life-threatening and limb-threatening injuries. She should be managed along lines promoted by the Advanced Trauma and Life Support (ATLS) system of care.

   She must receive supplemental oxygen to an unobstructed airway.

   A + C She should have her neck stabilized by in-line cervical immobilization techniques.
   B She should be able to breathe adequately.
   C She requires cardiovascular assessment and resuscitation.
   D She exhibits neurological disability which may change during the course of resuscitation.
   E She requires complete exposure and undressing, examination of her back by log-rolling and control of the environmental temperature to prevent cooling.

   Following this primary survey and simultaneous resuscitation she may prove stable enough to permit a secondary top-to-toe examination following application of ECG monitoring leads, pulse oximetry, urinary catheterization and consideration of the need for a gastric tube. Finally, definitive care will need to be carefully coordinated; this could require transfer to another institution for special investigations and neurosurgical input.

2. Bradycardia in the context of trauma and blood loss is an unusual observation. Normally the baroreceptors in the aortic arch and carotid sinus stimulate tachycardia with vasoconstriction to compensate for a falling blood pressure. A relative bradycardia may be observed in those with pre-existing heart block necessitating a cardiac pacemaker. It may also be encountered, as in this case, in those patients taking beta-adrenoceptor blocker therapy. It accompanies hypertension in those patients with critically raised intracranial pressure and is a feature of the autonomic neuropathy seen in high spinal injuries.

   Since the bradycardia complicates resuscitation it is sometimes necessary to institute invasive cardiovascular monitoring, for example, central venous or pulmonary arterial catheters earlier in the course of treatment. In fact this woman's vital signs responded promptly to the infusion of 1 l of synthetic colloid with the restoration of a pulse on the right hand. Her scalp wound was cleaned and packed by way of haemorrhage control. Nevertheless, her heart rate remained unchanged at 60 beats/min throughout the first hour of trauma care.

3. A trauma series of X-rays constitutes:
   (a) An adequate lateral C-spine vertebrae showing the base of the skull, all the cervical vertebrae and the cervicothoracic junction.
   (b) A chest X-ray.
   (c) A pelvic X-ray.

   In this patient the first lateral cervical film was inadequate and a 'swimmer's view' was taken to show all the vertebrae. An area of abnormality around the odontoid peg and her presenting paraplegia led to open-mouth views and thoracic vertebral and lumbar views following the secondary survey and after discussion with the regional neurosurgical unit. These X-rays in turn demonstrated abnormalities suggestive of vertebral collapse with displacement in the region of T4. Furthermore, the chest X-ray showed an isolated rib fracture of the fourth right rib with no associated pneumo- or haemothorax. The pelvic X-rays were normal.

   Arrangements were then completed for transfer to the regional neurosurgical unit for computed tomography (CT) or magnetic resonance imaging (MRI) scanning of head, cervical and thoracic vertebrae before further intervention.

4. The over-riding principle of initial care for the paraplegic patient is do no further harm. The patient must be log-rolled for care and caution exercised to pressure points in the now unfeeling limbs. It is also generally accepted that early reduction of fracture dislocations and immobilization can minimize neurological damage. Recent evidence also suggests that steroids may be of value in certain patients with incomplete spinal cord injuries. Their use should be determined in consultation with a neurosurgeon.

   In the acute phase it can be difficult to exclude intra-abdominal pathology. Peritoneal lavage is a useful diagnostic technique but interpretation can be complicated by retroperitoneal haematomata.

   Some patients develop discoordinated bowel activity with progressive abdominal distension and vomiting. The rectum must be emptied by about the fourth day after injury and this should be followed by regular evacuation on 3 days of the week so that over-distention of the bowel is avoided, a pattern of reflex evacuation established and faecal incontinence prevented. Similarly, although patients will require urethral or suprapubic bladder catheterization with continuous drainage, a regimen of intermittent catheterization may be instituted to encourage the return of reflex bladder function.

Prophylactic measures to minimize the risk of gastrointestinal haemorrhage and thromboembolic complications are essential, as are first-class nursing and physiotherapy to prevent pressure sores and fixed deformities. The ability to adjust skin blood flow and sweating is lost below the level of a complete spinal cord lesion and spinal-injury patients exhibit temperature control problems.

5. (a) The Revised Trauma Score (RTS) is a numerical score indicating severity of injury which can be calculated from Table 5.1. Adherence to these guidelines is thought to enhance interhospital transfer.

(b) The Injury Severity Score (ISS) is based on the Abbreviated Injury Score, a score on a numerical scale ranging from 1 (indicating minor injury) to 6 (virtually unsurvivable injury). An Abbreviated Injury Score is assigned to each of the six regions of the body: head or neck, face, chest, abdomen or pelvic contents, extremities and body surface. The ISS is defined as the sum of the squares of the Abbreviated Injury Severity scores for the three most severely injured body regions; see Trunkey (1991) for an example.

(c) The Acute Physiology and Chronic Health Evaluation (APACHE) scoring system is a widely applicable method for assessing severity of illness in the critically ill but not exclusively the critically injured. The APACHE II score consists of two parts: the acute physiology score, based on 12 measured variables and an assessment of the patient's previous state of health. Chronic health problems are scored for long-standing organ dysfunction and age. The impact of emergency surgery also attracts additional risk points. The final APACHE II score is the sum of the acute physiology, age and chronic health points calculated from the worst values during the first 24 h of intensive care. When the APACHE II

Table 5.1 Revised Trauma Score

	Variables	Score
A. Respiratory rate	10–24	4
(breaths/min)	25–35	3
	>/36	2
	1–9	1
	0	0
B. Systolic blood pressure	>89	4
(mmHg)	70–89	3
	50–69	2
	1–49	1
	0	0
C. Glasgow Coma Scale	13–15	4
score conversion	9–12	3
C = D + E + F	6–8	2
	4–5	1
	<4	0
D. Eye opening	Spontaneous	4
	To voice	3
	To pain	2
	None	1
E. Verbal response	Oriented	5
	Confused	4
	Inappropriate words	3
	Incomprehensible words	2
	None	1
F. Motor response	Obeys command	6
	Localizes pain	5
	Withdraw (pain)	4
	Flexion (pain)	3
	Extension (pain)	2
	None	1
Glasgow Coma Score	(Total D + E + F)	
Revised Trauma Score	Score = A + B + C	

score is weighted using previously defined coefficients assigned to specific diagnostic categories, there is a consistent relationship between APACHE II mortality predictions and observed hospital death rates throughout the spectrum from low to high risk of death.

References and further reading

Skinner D, Driscoll P and Earlam R (eds) (1991) *ABC of Major Trauma.* BMJ Publications, London

Trunkey D. (1991) Initial treatment of patients with extensive trauma. *New England Journal of Medicine* **324:** 1259–1263

J.D. Watson

Case 6 Pelvic trauma

A 27-year-old man was brought to casualty by ambulance following a fall from the third floor of a tower block. He was conscious and fully oriented, although his breath smelled of alcohol. The casualty officer achieved venous access with two 14-gauge cannulae and requested a full blood count and 10 units of group-specific blood. Cervical spine and chest radiographs were normal; however, the radiograph of the pelvis showed a clearly displaced fracture through the left pubic rami and disruption of the left sacroiliac joint. On examination he had a pulse of 120 beats/min and a blood pressure of 95/70 mmHg. His scrotum was severely bruised and swollen and a small amount of blood was present at the external penile meatus.

Questions

1. Outline the management of this patient's haemodynamic status.
2. What is the other injury suggested in association with the pelvic fracture, and how would you manage it?
3. Classify pelvic fractures and discuss their important differences and treatment.
4. What are the specific complications associated with pelvic fractures?

Answers

1. Pelvic fractures often present with massive invisible retroperitoneal haemorrhage and hypovolaemic shock; this remains the leading cause of mortality. A rapid assessment of the degree of shock is necessary and important information can be gained quickly by observing the skin, pulses, conscious level and both diastolic and systolic blood pressures. Once adequate venous access is achieved, initial fluid replacement should begin with 2 l of crystalloid, followed by either colloid solution or group-specific blood when available. Continual reassessment and response to intravenous fluid replacement is the key to the management of haemor-

rhage. A measurement of the urine output is essential and this should be facilitated by catheterization only following complete assessment of the genitourinary system. Central venous access via the internal jugular or subclavian route may be a valuable adjunct to management, particularly in the assessment of circulatory volume. This should not be a priority and detract from or delay other life-saving procedures.

If, despite aggressive fluid replacement, the patient remains haemodynamically unstable, then a further source of haemorrhage must be sought. Open diagnostic peritoneal lavage (DPL) should be performed above the umbilicus to avoid the haematoma that frequently extends from the pelvis into the lower abdominal wall. The haematoma may also leak into the free peritoneal cavity and the results must be interpreted carefully as approximately 15% of patients will have a false-positive result. If the DPL is *grossly* positive, i.e. >10 ml of blood aspirated from abdominal cavity prior to the infusion of 1 l of normal saline, then one must proceed to immediate laparotomy. If the DPL is *count*-positive only, i.e. >100 000 red blood cells per millilitre of drained fluid following the saline infusion, then one should proceed to stabilize the fracture with an external fixation device and delay the laparotomy. This has been shown significantly to reduce the blood requirement of patients with unstable pelvic fractures.

Pelvic angiography should be considered if available, as most persistent pelvic bleeding comes from branches of the internal iliac artery that are amenable to embolization. Arteriography will not only delineate the source of pelvic haemorrhage, but also exclude additional intra-abdominal sites of blood loss. The pneumatic antishock garment has been advocated by many trauma surgeons. However, this device has been shown to be inferior to external pelvic fixation and carries many potential complications if inappropriately used.

2. The other major injury described is urethral trauma and approximately 10% of pelvic fractures have associated urethral damage. The prostate is fixed to the pubic symphysis by puboprostatic ligaments and any severe disruption of the pubic symphysis may tear the prostate off the membranous urethra, which is attached to the pelvic floor. The membranous urethra below the prostate is therefore the usual site of

damage associated with pelvic fractures. Rupture is usually partial, but occasionally complete disruption and prosto-urethral dislocation occur. In the female the urethra is much more mobile and consequently less prone to injury.

These patients often have serious injuries and a urinary catheter is required to monitor urine output. It is therefore of great importance to make a rapid diagnosis and facilitate urine drainage. The signs of urethral injury caused by pelvic fracture are perineal bruising, blood at the external meatus and an inability to pass urine. In prostatourethral dislocation this may be accompanied by a high-riding prostate on rectal examination.

The investigation of choice is ascending urethrography using a water-soluble contrast medium. This not only confirms the rupture but also determines whether it is partial or complete. Full renal tract imaging is required to exclude any associated injury; intravenous urogram and/or ultrasound are the usual methods employed. Increasingly, computed tomography (CT) with enhancement is useful as it also allows an assessment of the bony injury, so that possible combined procedures of early pelvic fixation and urethral repair can be planned. However, it is often necessary to treat accompanying urinary tract injury, such as bladder perforation, before CT scanning can be performed.

The safest initial method of treatment is to pass a suprapubic catheter either percutaneously or by cystotomy if the bladder is not palpable or if the patient requires a laparotomy for other reasons. The definitive management of the urethral rupture is more controversial. Tension should *not* be applied to the bladder neck via traction on a balloon catheter as this may damage the sphincter. Partial ruptures should be managed conservatively and the resulting stricture dealt with at a later date. If prostourethral dislocation has occurred, early operative realignment is often advocated, holding the reduction by perineal tension sutures anchored to the anterior part of the prostatic capsule. A delayed procedure may alternatively be performed, rerouting the urethra anteriorly to join the prostate.

3. The pelvis is a semirigid osseoligamentous ring consisting of two iliac bones and the sacrum linked by strong ligaments. A fracture at one point in the ring is theoretically accompanied by disruption at a second point. This second break is often not visible, either because it reduces immedi-

ately or because the sacroiliac joints are only partially disrupted, the visible fracture is not displaced and the ring is stable. A fracture or joint disruption that is markedly displaced and all obvious double-ring fractures are unstable. Tile's widely used classification is based on the degree and

Table 6.1 Tile's classification of pelvic fractures

Type A – stable	
A1	Fractures not involving the ring
A2	Stable, minimally displaced fractures of the ring
Type B – rotationally unstable, vertically stable	
B1	Anterior–posterior compression fractures (open-book)
B2	Lateral compression: ipsilateral
B3	Lateral compression: contralateral
Type C – rotationally and vertically unstable	
C1	Unilateral
C2	Bilateral
C3	Associated with an acetabular fracture

type of instability present (Table 6.1).

(a) *Type A – stable:* This includes muscular avulsion fractures and minimally displaced ring fractures. Bedrest and analgesia is usually all that is required.

(b) *Type B – rotationally unstable, vertically stable:* Open-book injuries are commonly seen in patients who have fallen from a height directly on to the back of the pelvis, producing an anterior–posterior compression force. The ring fails both anteriorly, either at the symphysis or through two rami, and posteriorly, and as a consequence the pelvis opens out.

A lateral compression injury may apply an internal rotatory force causing fractures of the pubic rami or overlapping of the pubic bones. This is classically seen in patients who have been driven over by a motor vehicle. The posterior sacroiliac ligaments remain intact and the hemipelvis hinges around them.

(c) *Type C – rotationally and vertically unstable:* There is disruption of the ring at two levels or more and particularly of the strong posterior ligaments with vertical displacement of one or both sides of the pelvis.

Patients with type B and C fractures are usually multiply injured and the mortality is very high. There is often associated pelvic visceral or neurovascular damage to the lower limb. The most efficient way of achieving and maintaining a reduction is by the application of an external fixator with pins in both iliac blades connected by an anterior bar. This will also help control the degree of haemorrhage by reducing the volume of the pelvic cavity and producing a tamponade effect on the viscera. Bedrest is mandatory for 8–10 weeks and, if there is an element of vertical instability, this should be combined with lower-limb traction. If reduction has not been achieved, then it may be possible internally to reduce and fix the fracture with a combination of devices. Such operations are hazardous and should only be attempted at specialized centres. Although fractures of the acetabulum may also be ring fractures, involvement of the joint raises special problems and they are considered separately. Any dislocation needs to be reduced and the lower limb put in traction until a CT can be performed and fixation planned if necessary. Further classification describes the anatomical relationship of the fracture within the acetabulum.

4. (a) *Immediate*
   (i) Haemorrhage.
   (ii) Genitourinary injury – second only to urethral injury, traumatic rupture of the bladder is a common complication. The physical signs may be minimal and a cystogram is performed to delineate the injury. However, CT with contrast has many advantages as it allows displacement by large haematomas to be distinguished from rupture.
   (iii) Nerve injury – the lumbar and sacral plexi are at risk from posterior pelvic injuries together with the sciatic nerve, from hip dislocation and acetabular fractures, and the femoral and obturator nerves as they leave the pelvis. Full neurological examination is essential in all pelvic injuries.
   (iv) Vascular injury – this is not only to the branches of the internal iliac vessels within the pelvis, but also the external iliac and femoral artery which may compromise the perfusion of the lower limb.
   (v) Bowel injury – the sigmoid colon, with its mesentery, is a mobile structure and therefore not readily injured in pelvic fracture. The rectum and anal canal are more firmly tethered to the urogenital

structures and muscular floor of the pelvis and consequently at greater risk. Rectal examination is, therefore, mandatory in any patient suspected of pelvic injury.

(vi) Vaginal injury – bony fragments can perforate the lining, similar to the rectum, and a vaginal examination must always be performed.

(b) *Delayed*

(i) Iliofemoral venous thrombosis is common in patients confined to bedrest for long periods.

(ii) Secondary osteoarthritis may occur in the sacroiliac and hip joints. Acetabular fractures present a significant problem as the joint is disrupted and the articular cartilage often damaged, resulting in malcongruent loading and secondary osteoarthritis. This may ultimately require joint replacement.

(iii) Myositis ossificans is common after severe soft-tissue injury and extensive surgical procedures.

(iv) Malunion is common but does not usually present significant problems except in females of child-bearing age. Caesarean section may be required for delivery.

Further reading

ATLS Course Manual 1988. American College of Surgeons, Chicago

Paul A. Harris
Peter Baird

Case 7 Principles of donor management

A 38-year-old female suddenly collapsed at work having complained of a severe frontal headache. She was admitted to hospital with a Glasgow Coma Score of 3 and bilateral dilated non-reacting pupils. Computed tomography (CT) scan revealed massive subarachnoid haemorrhage. The patient was admitted to the intensive care unit and ventilated and invasively monitored. Her neurological status remained unchanged and brainstem death was confirmed after 24 h. The patient's family expressed a wish that she might become an organ donor. During preparation for organ donation, her urine output fell despite an adequate blood pressure. Later her blood pressure also started to fall. The plasma sodium rose to 173 mmol/l with an osmolality of 329 mmol/kg. Oxygenation remained adequate with an FIo_2 of 35%, but active rewarming was required to maintain the patient's temperature above 35°C.

Questions

1. How would you initially treat the fall in urine output?
2. Why does the blood pressure fall? What treatment would you institute and what cardiovascular monitoring is required?
3. Why does the plasma sodium rise and how may it be corrected?
4. What precautions must be taken if lung donation is planned?
5. Why is the patient at risk of becoming hypothermic?

Answers

1. A fall in urine output may reflect inadequate intravascular filling. Intravenous fluids should be administered if the central venous pressure is low. In the presence of adequate perfusion and central venous pressures, a low-dose dopamine infusion (2 μg/kg per min) should be initiated. A donor urine output of less than 80 ml/h prior to organ harvest is associated with a higher incidence of tubular necrosis in the transplanted kidneys. It is therefore essential to maintain an adequate urine output during this critical period. Small

incremental intravenous doses of frusemide (10 mg) may be given if low-dose dopamine fails to produce a diuresis.

2. Immediately following brainstem death, there is a period of high sympathetic activity with hypertension and the risk of cardiac arrhythmias. Following this, however, there is loss of sympathetic tone and profound vasodilatation which causes the hypotension seen in this patient. This is aggravated by an associated myocardial depression and the possibility of hypovolaemia. Hypotension should initially be treated with aggressive fluid replacement to maintain central venous pressure at supranormal levels. Inotropes are indicated in those who failed to respond to volume expansion. Dopamine is used initially because of its vasodilator effects on renal and mesenteric vessels at low infusion rates. The requirement for high-dose inotropic support is indicative of myocardial failure and dobutamine should be added if the requirements for dopamine exceed $5\,\mu g/kg$ per min. Although dobutamine will increase cardiac output, its beta-mediated peripheral dilatory effects may worsen the hypotension and agents such as adrenaline or noradrenaline may be required.

It has recently been appreciated that marked endocrine dysfunction may contribute to the cardiovascular instability following brainstem death. Loss of anterior pituitary function causes a fall in T_3 which leads to inhibition of mitochondrial function and a subsequent deterioration in myocardial function. Many units now use hormone infusion as an aid to cardiovascular support and a means of reducing inotrope requirements. Thyroxine (T_4/T_3), pitressin (antidiuretic hormone) and insulin are the agents most commonly used in this respect.

ECG, direct arterial blood pressure, central venous pressure, urine output and temperature monitoring are mandatory in all potential organ donors. In those with cardiovascular instability and a requirement for inotropic support, a pulmonary artery catheter should be inserted to allow monitoring of pulmonary capillary wedge pressure and cardiac output.

3. Posterior pituitary function is also lost following brainstem death. This results in diabetes insipidus, characterized by an inappropriate diuresis, hypovolaemia, hyperosmolality and hypernatraemia. Volume replacement with 5% dextrose may initially return plasma sodium levels to normal and this

may be supplemented with water via a nasogastric tube. Severe diabetes insipidus however requires treatment with vasopressin (DDAVP). This drug causes a dose-dependent vasoconstriction which is associated with tubular necrosis and decreased renal graft survival. Current opinion favours the use of vasopressin administered as a constant low-dose infusion (0.5 units/h) to reduce urine output to 1.5–3 ml/kg per h.

4. Meticulous attention to aseptic technique, particularly during endotracheal suction, will minimize the risk of pulmonary infection. The inspired oxygen concentration must be maintained at a level high enough to ensure adequate saturation of haemoglobin, but if the lungs are to be transplanted the FIo_2 should not exceed 60% to avoid the risks of pulmonary oxygen toxicity. Modest levels of positive end-expiratory pressure (about $5\,cmH_2O$) will prevent alveolar collapse without having deleterious effects on cardiac output. The transplant team will wish to see a recent chest X-ray.

5. A fall in body temperature is common after brainstem death because temperature regulation is markedly impaired. There is a reduction in heat production secondary to a fall in metabolic rate, loss of muscular activity and peripheral vasodilatation. Although mild hypothermia may offer some protection to organs to be transplanted, temperatures below 32°C result in decreased myocardial performance and coagulopathies. Furthermore, brainstem death cannot be diagnosed if the core temperature is less than 35°C. Active warming with the use of space blankets and warmed intravenous fluids is often required after brainstem death.

Further reading

Hill SA and Park GR. (1990) Management of multiple organ donors. Intensive care developments and controversies. *Ballieres Clinical Anaesthesiology* **4**: 587–605

Robertson KM and Ryan Cook D. (1990) Perioperative management of the multiorgan donor. *Anesthesia and Analgesia* **70**: 546–556

Soifer BE and Gelb AW. (1989) The multiple organ donor: identification and management. *Annals of Internal Medicine* **110**: 814–823

Timmins AC and Hinds CJ. (1991) Management of the multiple-organ donor. *Current Opinion in Anaesthesiology* **4**: 287–292

Martin Smith and Claire Hornick

Case 8   Lung cancer

A 63-year-old smoker attended his general practitioner for persistent cough that he felt he had been unable to shake off over the Christmas holidays. Despite the food available over the festive season, his appetite was poor and he had noticed half a stone (about 3 kg) in weight loss over the previous 6–8 weeks. Recently his sputum had been a little blood-streaked.

The patient's doctor referred him for a chest X-ray which showed a 4 cm spiculated opacity in the upper right lung.

Questions

1. What is the likely diagnosis?
2. How is the tumour classified pathologically?
3. How else may this disease present?
4. What further investigations should be carried out?
5. What treatment options are available for this patient?
6. When is surgery indicated?
7. What surgical options may be considered?

Answers

1. Lung cancer.
2. There are three major pathological types of lung cancer. About one-half of the cancers presenting are squamous cell carcinoma, 13% adenocarcinoma and a further 13% are small cell carcinoma (also known as oat cell carcinoma). Large cell carcinomas occur in 10% of presentations.
3. Lung cancer may present due to the effects of the primary tumour and its invasion locally, which may include a hoarse voice (recurrent laryngeal nerve palsy), pericardial effusion, brachial plexus pain or loss of muscle power in the arm (Pancoast tumour). The effects of secondary tumour include cerebral symptoms and signs and bone pain and the systemic effects of a cancer include weight loss, lassitude, fatigue and loss of appetite.

Certain kinds of lung cancer may cause endocrine symptoms and hypertrophic osteoarthropathy is also associated with lung cancer. Four out of five lung cancers are associated with tobacco smoking and prevention through education is probably the most important part of management of this disease. Radioactivity, asbestos, chromium or nickel exposure, coal gas and radon gas have also been associated with this disease.

4. Once the diagnosis is suspected, usually on chest X-ray, attention must be directed not only to the overall condition of the patient but also to specifically finding the stage and type of the cancer as on this the treatment instituted and prognosis will depend. The patient should have blood tests, including a full blood count, urea and electrolytes and liver function tests and radiology, including a computed tomogram (CT) of the chest, with special attention being focused on the presence or absence of enlarged mediastinal nodes. A bronchoscopy must be carried out to see the extent of intrabronchial tumour, to biopsy it, to find the histological type or to take washings with cytological examination if the tumour is not biopsiable. Lung function tests should be done in order to see the respiratory reserve, particularly if surgery is considered. Sputum cytology can be important in order to find the histological type and sometimes to check for tuberculosis infection. A needle biopsy (under radiographic screening) of the tumour mass may be indicated to give histological diagnosis.

5. The treatment of a patient with lung cancer should be considered in three ways: prevention, cure, which hinges particularly on early diagnosis and the type and stage of the cancer, and palliation, which unfortunately is the treatment needed for many patients.

   The treatment may consist of surgery, radiotherapy or chemotherapy.

   Radiotherapy may be indicated to try to obtain cure in early non-small cell cancers that have not spread but is usually most often used for palliation, particularly for superior vena cava obstruction, pain, haemoptysis, dyspnoea or recurrent cough. Chemotherapy is primarily indicated in small cell carcinoma and at the present time is not usually the treatment of choice for other types of lung cancer.

6. Surgery is indicated in a patient with good lung function (usually considered to be an FEV_1 of greater than 1 l in 1 s)

with non-small cell carcinoma in whom the cancer has not spread beyond the hemithorax. Staging of the lung cancer is usually the TNM classification – T standing for tumour, N for nodes and M for metastases. The T classification is T_1–T_4. T_1 is a small tumour less than 3 cm with no invasion proximal to a lobar bronchus. T_2 is a larger tumour, greater than 3 cm but not within 2 cm of the main carina. T_3 is when the tumour has spread to the chest wall, pericardium, mediastinal pleura or diaphragm and T_4 one that has spread to the heart, great vessels, oesophagus, main carina or the vertebral bodies. Nodes are classified as N_1–N_3. N_1 is when the hilar nodes are involved, N_2 the mediastinal nodes and N_3 the contralateral nodes within the chest, supraclavicular or scalene nodes. Metastases may be either M_0 (no distant metastases) or M_1 (distant metastases present). The staging preoperatively of a lung cancer should be accurate and is a good indication of the prognosis.

Surgery is indicated in T_1 and T_2 tumours and some T_3 tumours. Surgery is helpful in N_1 tumours and in some N_2 tumours but not N_3 tumours. Obviously surgery is not indicated if there are distant metastases.

The critical issue is whether lymph nodes are involved with tumour and if so, where they are. This can usually be determined on CT scan but operative biopsy of the lymph nodes through a mediastinoscopy or mediastinotomy may be indicated in special circumstances.

There are currently more than 30 000 deaths per year in the UK from lung cancer. Small cell carcinoma has a uniformly poor prognosis with a mean survival time of less than 3 months. If the patient can be operated on, then overall 5-year survival is 20–35%. If the patient has no nodes involved and a tumour which is not invading beyond the lung then the 5-year prognosis with surgery is greater than 60%. However, if the nodes in the hilum are involved then the 5-year prognosis for tumours confined to the lung may be as low as 40% and if the mediastinum is involved, 30%.

7. Surgical treatment consists of lung resection. This is either a lobectomy if the tumour is small and confined to the lung, or a pneumonectomy. This should be associated with a lymph node dissection at the hilum and often within the mediastinum. For N_3 tumours invading outside the lung but into the major mediastinal structures, then resection of the chest wall or the pericardium can be carried out successfully. The

hospital mortality for a lobectomy in the UK is currently approximately 2% and for a pneumonectomy 5–6%.

Further reading

Shields TW. (1989) General thoracic surgery. In: *Carcinoma of the Lung*, pp. 890–934. Lea & Febiger, Philadelphia

Peter Smith

Case 9 Peripheral vascular disease

A man aged 62 had developed pain in his right foot at rest and particularly at night. This had persisted for 2 weeks and was resulting in considerable loss of sleep. There was a history of pain in the left calf on walking for about 100 m during the previous 6 months.

Examination revealed that pulses were absent in both feet and the right foot was cold and pale compared with the left. There was a right carotid bruit.

Questions

1. What is the likely diagnosis? What other bedside tests should be carried out?
2. What investigations are appropriate?
3. How will you be influenced by the carotid bruit?
4. Describe the treatment options that need to be considered.
5. What follow-up arrangements should be made?

Answers

1. The likely diagnosis is that this patient has vascular rest pain due to occlusive arterial disease. The previous history of pain in the left calf on walking, likely to be vascular claudication, also suggests that this patient is an arteriopath, as does the presence of carotid bruits. Vascular rest pain is usually severe and relentless and the patient may report obtaining some relief by hanging the leg out of bed or by sleeping upright in a chair. As well as ascertaining the precise details of the pain, a full history should be obtained with reference to cardiac and respiratory disease, smoking history and a history of diabetes.

   In addition a full clinical examination must be performed with particular attention to the presence or absence of the femoral pulses and the presence or absence of femoral or iliac bruits. Aneurysms of the aorta, femoral and popliteal arteries should be sought as emboli from these sources can result in similar symptoms. Other clinical tests include looking for delayed capillary refill time and Buerger's test, which consists of looking for pallor on elevation and rubor on dependence.

The other bedside test of great value is to measure the patient's Doppler foot pressures. This is done by finding the dorsalis pedis and posterior tibial pulses using a hand-held Doppler probe. A sphygmomanometer cuff is then inflated around the lower calf and the pressure at which the signal disappears is taken as the systolic pressure in that vessel. The pressures are then related to the brachial systolic pressure as the ankle:brachial index, e.g. ankle pressure 60 mmHg, brachial pressure 120 mmHg = index of 0.5.

The Fontaine classification (Table 9.1) allows the grading of limb ischaemia on clinical grounds. According to this classification this patient is Fontaine stage III. This clinical classification has been supplemented by definitions which may include the Doppler pressures. One of the most widely accepted defines critical limb ischaemia (i.e. ischaemia which endangers the limb or part of the limb) as persistently recurring rest pain requiring analgesia for longer than 2 weeks and/or ulceration gangrene of the foot or toes plus an ankle systolic pressure of less than 50 mmHg. One must be aware, however, that calcification of the arteries (especially common in diabetes) may make measurement of the ankle pressures unreliable. In these patients measurements

Table 9.1 Fontaine classification of limb ischaemia

Stage	Symptoms/signs
I	No clinical symptoms
II	Intermittent claudication
III	Ischaemic rest pain
IV	Ischaemic ulcer, gangrene

of the degree of elevation of the limb required for the Doppler signal to disappear may be more reliable.

2. Patients presenting with critical limb ischaemia require prompt investigation and treatment. Test urine for sugar. Resting ECG, chest X-ray, full blood count and group, erythrocyte sedimentation rate, serum creatinine, electrolytes,

liver function tests and clotting screen should be carried out on all patients. If there is ulceration or necrosis swabs should be sent for bacteriology and plain X-rays or bone scan to look for evidence of osteomyelitis may also be helpful.

When indicated, patients may require further assessment of cardiac or respiratory disease. This is particularly so if aortic surgery is planned, when occasional patients may benefit from prior coronary artery bypass or angioplasty. It should be remembered that, because of decreased activity patients with critical limb ischaemia may not report angina or shortness of breath on exertion. Respiratory function tests, blood-gas analysis, stress echocardiography, stress cardiac nuclide scan, estimation of ejection fraction or coronary angiography may be helpful in some patients.

Angiography is the most important investigation for defining the anatomy of the arterial occlusive disease and for planning subsequent management. Angiography can be performed by either intravenous or intra-arterial injection. Intravenous injection is less invasive but produces poorer-quality pictures, especially in patients with poor cardiac outputs. Most centres now rely on digital subtraction techniques to produce the highest-quality images. When intra-arterial angiography is being performed it is best if angioplasty (when feasible) be performed on the same occasion to prevent the potential morbidity of a second arterial puncture. This requires a close working relationship between the vascular surgeon and radiologist.

Other tests which may be of some value include duplex scanning, Doppler waveform analysis performed at segmental levels in the limb, direct femoral pressure measurements to aid assessment of aortoiliac disease and laser Doppler or oxygen electrode assessment of the microcirculation. These tests, however, only rarely alter management decision based on angiography and clinical assessment.

3. As part of the history, symptoms suggestive of transient ischaemic attacks should be sought. If there is a history suggestive of symptoms attributable to a carotid stenosis then further investigation is indicated. This would usually include duplex scan of the carotid arteries, angiography and either computed tomography or magnetic resonance imaging of the brain. A neurological opinion should also be obtained. There is now good evidence that symptomatic

carotid stenosis of greater than 70% should be treated by carotid endarterectomy in patients with a reasonable life expectancy. In this patient a decision to perform a carotid endarterectomy and its timing would need to be decided in relation to the degree of limb ischaemia, the type of peripheral arterial surgery planned and the patient's general condition.

If there are no symptoms attributable to the carotid stenosis then the evidence that carotid endarterectomy is helpful prior to reconstructive arterial surgery is much less clear. It is probably reasonable to assess the degree of stenosis by duplex scanning but to consider intervention only if there are bilateral high-grade stenoses in a patient who requires major aortic reconstruction or coronary bypass. Otherwise, the carotid bruit should be ignored at this stage but should be flagged up as a likely marker of coronary artery disease.

4. The treatment options to be considered include surgical reconstruction, percutaneous angioplasty, medical management and amputation. Which of these will be appropriate will in a large part be determined by the results of angiography which will show whether bypass grafting or angioplasty is technically possible. Other factors to be considered are the patient's fitness to undergo major surgery and prospects for subsequent mobilization.

Percutaneous balloon angioplasty carries a lower morbidity and mortality than surgical reconstruction. It may be applicable in patients unfit for surgery or as an adjunct to surgery since the majority of patients with critical limb ischaemia will have occlusions at more than one level. For example, an iliac lesion may be dilated prior to a femoropopliteal bypass graft.

When critical ischaemia has worsened suddenly then it may be due to thrombosis on a pre-existing stenosis and it may be worthwhile considering thrombolysis. A thrombolytic agent such as streptokinase, tissue plasminogen activator (t-PA) or urokinase is given by direct arterial infusion. After lysis of an occlusion which would have required surgical bypass, a lesion suitable for angioplasty may be revealed.

Reconstructive surgery is indicated when there is no such lesion and when there is sufficient run-off. The reconstruction required will depend on the anatomy of the occlusions or stenoses as revealed by angiography. An important principle is to deal with the more proximal lesions first if they are believed to be haemodynamically significant.

Primary amputation is indicated where angiography shows that no reconstruction is possible or when the patient has no prospect of walking such as if he or she has already developed a major fixed flexion at the hip or knee or has had a disabling stroke. In other cases amputation may be preferable to subjecting a sick patient to repeated surgical procedures with little chance of success. This is often the case after initial attempt at bypass grafting has failed. Below-knee amputation is preferred to above-knee as more patients will subsequently be able to mobilize on a prosthetic limb. When reconstruction is not possible and immediate amputation is not required, some patients may respond to conservative and medical therapy. Correctable factors such as heart failure, anaemia or polycythaemia, dehydration and infection should be treated. There is little evidence that anticoagulation is of value but vasodilators or prostaglandin analogues may help, as may lumbar sympathectomy, which in addition may reduce the degree of pain felt by the patient.

5. The follow-up required will depend on the treatment that the patient has undergone. After amputation follow-up may be best carried out by the patient's general practitioner or limb-fitting centre. Routine clinic follow-up will be required for those who have had aortic surgery or angioplasty. If an infrainguinal graft has been performed then graft surveillance should be carried out. Failure of grafts below the inguinal ligament in the first months after surgery is usually due to technical errors or because there is very poor run-off. Failures after 1 year are mostly due to progression of disease. Failures in the middle period are, however, in the main due to the development of stenosis caused by intimal hyperplasia leading then to thrombosis. If identified, such a stenosis can be dealt with by angioplasty or revisional surgery. The best method of detecting these stenoses before they cause occlusions is by duplex scanning (non-invasive) or angiography (invasive) at intervals during the first year following surgery.

Further reading

Bell, PRF, Jamieson CW and Ruckley CV. (1991) *Surgical Management of Vascular Disease*. WB Saunders, London

Dormandy JA and Stock G. (1990) *Critical Leg Ischaemia – Its Pathophysiology and Management*. Springer-Verlag, Berlin

Eastcott HHG. (1992) *Arterial Surgery*, 3rd edn. Churchill Livingstone, Edinburgh

Rutherford RB. (1994) *Vascular Surgery*. WB Saunders, Philadelphia

Averil O. Mansfield
Gerard Stansby

Case 10   Ischaemic lower limb

A 70-year-old man was admitted with acute pain in the right
leg of several hours' duration. He gave a history of stable exer-
tional angina and had smoked 20 cigarettes a day for many
years. On direct questioning, he admitted to pain in both legs
on walking for some months, which was worse on the right. On
examination, the right leg was colder than the left and the foot
and toes showed dusky purple disoloration with slow capillary
return. The pulses in the right leg were impalpable below the
femoral. Movement and sensation were normal.

Questions

1. What is the diagnosis?
2. Which investigations would you perform?
3. How would you treat the patient further?
4. Which types of treatment are available?
5. What are the contraindications to this type of treatment?
6. What are the complications?

Answers

1. Arterial thrombosis in the right leg, most likely of the superficial femoral or popliteal artery secondary to underlying
   atherosclerosis, causing preceding intermittent claudication.
2. The leg is not critically ischaemic with no sensorimotor loss
   and hence does not require emergency surgery. Lower-
   limb arteriography should be performed with progression
   to thrombolysis if appropriate.
   Varying angiographic techniques are available. The commonest is to perform diagnostic angiography using a 5F pig-
   tail catheter inserted via the contralateral femoral artery.
   The catheter is positioned in the lower abdominal aorta and
   angiograms of both legs are obtained, preferably using
   non-ionic contrast media.
   The angiogram demonstrated patent right iliac and
   common femoral arteries. The right superficial femoral
   artery showed atheromatous disease with distal occlusion
   just above the level of the adductor canal. Run-off into the

calf was poor, with a few collateral vessels reconstituting a faint posterior tibial artery.

3. The patient is suitable for thrombolysis treatment providing there are no contraindications. This can either be performed from the contralateral side by passing a catheter over the aortic bifurcation or by performing an ipsilateral antegrade femoral artery puncture. The catheter tip is advanced to the level of the thrombus and, if possible, a guidewire passed into the thrombus to help disrupt the thrombus and increase the surface area amenable to lysis. The thrombus may be lysed from the distal end in a retrograde manner or antegradely from the proximal end. Thrombolysis may be performed as a low-dose infusion regime or more recently as a 'pulse-spray' technique, using higher doses over a shorter time. Thrombus aspiration is sometimes used to accelerate the procedure. This is performed from the ipsilateral groin with a catheter via a percutaneous access sheath.

4. Agents used for thrombolysis are streptokinase, tissue plasminogen activator (rt-PA) and urokinase.

   (a) Streptokinase: This has been widely used for thrombolysis and is the cheapest agent available. However, it is antigenic and therefore cannot be used for repeat thrombolysis within at least 6 months, and it has been reported that antibodies to streptokinase may persist for up to 5 years.

   (b) rt-PA: Now widely used for thrombolysis and regarded by many as more effective than streptokinase. This increased efficacy may be associated with more haemorrhagic complications. rt-PA is not allergenic or pyrogenic. It remains significantly more expensive than streptokinase.

   (c) Urokinase: First isolated from human urine in 1946, urokinase has been used extensively for thrombolysis in the USA and Europe but not in the UK.

   These agents may be used as either a low-dose or high-dose local infusion. Low-dose infusion uses streptokinase 5000–10 000 units/h, rt-PA 0.5–1.0 mg/h or urokinase 50 000–100 000 units/h. High-dose infusion regimes involve injecting large boluses of the agent, e.g. rt-PA 5 mg or urokinse 250 000 units every 10 min. A modification of this technique is the pulse-spray method. A long multiple-side-hole catheter is either embedded in the thrombus or a tip-occluding guidewire is inserted and repeated small doses of thrombolysis are injected frequently; lysis is achieved in 1–2 h. Typically, rt-PA 20 mg or urokinase 1 million units may be injected.

The patient responded well to an infusion of rt-PA to reveal critical stenoses in the distal superficial femoral and popliteal arteries. A good angiographic result was seen following angioplasty of these lesions.

5. The time that may be involved in thrombolysis, particularly the low-dose infusion regimes, must be considered before treatment is commenced. If the limb is severely ischaemic, surgery is probably more appropriate. Severe ischaemia with loss of motor function is a contraindication to thrombolysis due to the length of time to successful lysis and the increased risk of myoglobin and other metabolites being released into the circulation following restoration of arterial flow.

Recent haemorrhage, particularly a recent haemorrhagic stroke, is a contraindication to thrombolysis. Relative contraindications include recent major surgery, peptic ulceration or gastrointestinal bleeding, uncontrolled hypertension, generalized bleeding diathesis and haemorrhagic diabetic retinopathy. The benefit of thrombolysis must be carefully considered against the risk of bleeding in these cases.

6. Haemorrhage is the most serious complication of thrombolysis. Haematoma or bleeding at the arterial puncture site may be controlled by compression. If bleeding cannot be easily controlled, thrombolysis should be discontinued and a full clotting screen obtained. Major haemorrhage requiring transfusion or surgery has been reported in up to 5% of cases but this figure is lower with shorter, high-dose thrombolysis regimes. Cryoprecipitate or fresh frozen plasma may be used to reverse the action of the thrombolysis, but may need to be repeated and careful attention must be paid to the coagulation profile. If the patient becomes hypotensive without obvious signs of bleeding, retroperitoneal haemorrhage should be considered (or anaphylaxis if streptokinase or urokinase has been given).

Distal embolization of thrombus during thrombolysis is reported in approximately 9% of cases and is due to the clot softening and breaking up. The patient may suffer increased pain with worsening of the ischaemia and thrombolysis must not be stopped but continued, and the dose of the thrombolytic agent increased if possible to ensure rapid lysis of the distal emboli. This is usually successful and surgery is rarely required unless the limb is critically ischaemic. Surgery in this situation is however technically difficult as the calf run-off vessels are occluded by thrombus. Death from local thrombolysis is now rare and is usually due to either major haemorrhage or revascularization syndrome.

Further reading

Gaines PA and Beard JD. (1991) Radiological management of acute lower limb ischaemia. *British Journal of Hospital Medicine* **45:** 343–353

Plant G. (1994) Consensus in thrombolysis. *Journal of Interventional Radiology* **9:** 47–56

Claire Cousins

Case 11   Cerebral vascular disease

A 72-year-old female smoker presented to her family doctor with a minor stroke (right arm/leg hemisensory and motor loss with dysphasia). Blood pressure was 140/75 mmHg. She was noted to have bilateral carotid bruits, the right being harsher than the left. She was admitted to hospital and, although she made a rapid recovery, she still had slight right arm weakness and a clumsy hand 10 days after onset. A computed tomography (CT) scan revealed a small area of infarction within the left middle cerebral artery territory and duplex ultrasound scanning demonstrated bilateral severe carotid disease. On the left side the stenosis was probably greater than 70% (clear view obscured by acoustic shadowing from a calcified plaque) with distal extension above the limits of the ultrasound scan. On the right side, the stenosis was 90% but limited to the proximal 2 cm of the internal carotid artery.

Questions

1. What management advice would you offer to this patient?
2. What factors in the history might influence the timing of any operation?
3. How might surgical access to distal carotid disease be achieved and what risks are increased?
4. What monitoring or cerebral protection facilities might be used to avoid complications?
5. What advice would you offer with regard to the asymptomatic right carotid stenosis?
6. Does serial surveillance imaging influence management decisions postoperatively?

Answers

1. This patient has suffered a left carotid territory stroke with a residual neurological deficit. Ultrasound suggests severe bilateral stenoses. The first line of management is correction of risk factors (smoking) and starting aspirin. Because she probably has a severe symptomatic stenosis, the risks of carotid endarterectomy should be discussed. Provided that

she accepts these risks, the next line of management is carotid angiography because of the inability of the duplex scan to image above the plaque and to determine the true degree of stenosis because of acoustic shadowing.

2. Patients presenting with a stroke and particularly those with a residual neurological deficit are at higher risk of suffering a perioperative neurological complication than others. Accordingly, many surgeons would recommend delaying carotid surgery until 6 weeks had elapsed following the acute event. This increased susceptibility may be due to the increased risk of overlying plaque thrombus being present during the first 4 weeks after the event, haemorrhagic transformation of the infarct following reperfusion, impaired cerebral autoregulation in the vicinity of the infarct, and the absence of an established collateral circulation. There are however ongoing studies to assess the safety and efficacy of surgery in the acute post-stroke period because it is accepted from the natural history of stroke that the risk of a further event is also higher during this time period.

3. Distal extension of the carotid plaque into the higher reaches of the internal carotid artery occurs in about 5% of symptomatic patients and increases the risk of perioperative stroke and cranial nerve injury.

   Access to the middle aspect of the internal carotid artery can be facilitated by asking the anaesthetist to use nasotracheal (as opposed to orotracheal) intubation plus division of the posterior belly of digastric. This then significantly widens the apex of the access triangle between the mandible and sternomastoid. More distal access can be achieved by division of the styloid process with or without bilateral mandibular subluxation (requiring intra- and postoperative interdental arch bar fixation) or temporary ipsilateral mandibular subluxation. In the latter technique, the wires and pins are removed at the end of the operation and the patient is allowed to eat the next day.

4. There are a large number of intraoperative monitoring methods, although no uniform policy as to their effectiveness. This remains the case despite awareness that thromboembolism, rather than haemodynamic failure, is the most important cause of operative morbidity and that technical error is the commonest cause of thromboembolism. Temporary shunt deployment is probably more a matter of

personal preference as there is currently no definitive evidence that it reduces morbidity.

Simple methods to evaluate the adequacy of cerebral perfusion after carotid clamping include stump pressure and a subjective assessment of carotid backflow. However, these only provide a one-off assessment and no further information during the rest of the procedure. Most importantly, a high stump pressure will not prevent a stroke caused by embolism due to technical error. The more complex methods (continuous electroencephalogram and sensory evoked potentials) require considerable technical support and expertise and are rarely used in the UK. This is probably because of the perception that, although capable of detecting cerebral dysfunction, they are too expensive to operate and there is usually not much that can be done to correct the abnormality once it has occurred.

There is however a trend towards employing continuous transcranial Doppler (TCD) monitoring throughout the procedure with or without complete angioscopic examination of the endarterectomized zone. TCD provides instantaneous information on blood-flow velocity in the ipsilateral middle cerebral artery, shunt malfunction and kinking, intraoperative emboli and perioperative carotid thrombosis. Completion angioscopy is performed through the arteriotomy prior to restoration of flow in order to identify residual stenoses, mural thrombus and intimal flaps. Its principal advantage is that any defects can be corrected before restoring flow to the brain. Other assessment or quality control methods include near infrared spectroscopic measurement of cerebral oxygenation, continuous-wave Doppler waveform assessment and colour-flow imaging.

5. The simplest answer is that no one really knows what to advise with regard to patients referred with an asymptomatic stenosis. Two multicentre trials have published inconclusive results; the European Asymptomatic Carotid Surgery Trial is ongoing while the American Asymptomatic Carotid Artery Study has published limited interim data following intervention by the monitoring committee. In the latter, the principal points to note were a low annual risk of ipsilateral stroke (0.5%) following surgery as compared with 2% per annum for medically treated patients. However, the long-term surgical stroke risk does not include

perioperative morbidity (a creditable 2.3% in this study). In short, about 20 asymptomatic patients with severe carotid stenoses must undergo carotid endarterectomy in order to prevent one having a stroke over the next 5 years. As a result of these rather inconclusive data, most UK surgeons would still prefer either to avoid operating on asymptomatic stenoses such as that described in the case report or to include them in the ongoing European study. In the end, it is likely that a meta-analysis of all randomized studies will be necessary to provide definitive advice.

6. At present there is no evidence that serially imaging the carotid arteries of patients following carotid endarterectomy (with duplex ultrasound or intravenous digital subtraction angiography (IVDSA)) alters clinical management. In particular, it does not appear to prevent late stroke. Following endarterectomy, the average annual risk of stroke in the operated artery territory is about 1.8% (this also includes the perioperative risk) and is approximately 1.4% in the contralateral non-operated artery. More importantly, late strokes are not usually preceded by an antecedent transient ischaemic attack (thus negating the role of regular clinical review) and many have no evidence of significant disease recurrence or progression (thereby compromising the role of surveillance imaging). It is probably therefore appropriate to discharge patients after their first postoperative review with instructions to return should any new symptoms arise.

Further reading

Greenhalgh RM and Hollier L. (eds) (1993) *Surgery for Stroke*. WB Saunders, London
Naylor AR, Bell PRF and Ruckley CN. (1992) Monitoring and cerebral protection during carotid endarterectomy. *British Journal of Surgery* **79**: 735–741

A. Ross Naylor

Case 12   Monitoring the critically ill patient

A 60-year-old woman is admitted with an acute abdomen for a laparotomy. Medical problems include left ventricular failure and angina treated with frusemide and diltiazam respectively. Preoperative investigations are essentially normal, although the urea and creatinine are both raised and the ECG indicates left ventricular hypertrophy and anterior ischaemia. Uncomplicated bowel resection is performed for perforation of a diverticulum with evidence of faecal peritonitis. Intraoperatively there was cardiovascular instability and an episode of supraventricular tachycardia requiring treatment.

Questions

1. Where do you think the patient should be cared for post-operatively and why?
2. What monitoring is appropriate for the patient?
3. List the sites and complications for (a) invasive arterial blood pressure and (b) central venous pressure (CVP) monitoring.
4. Describe an accepted cannulation procedure for the right internal jugular vein.
5. If inotropic agents are required, what additional monitoring would you prefer?
6. What information does this extra monitoring supply and what are the complications associated with its use?

Answers

1. The patient should be transferred to the intensive care unit postoperatively. The high mortality rate associated with a faecal peritonitis and the likelihood that other organ systems may be affected means that intensive monitoring and organ support will be required. The pre-existing renal and cardiovascular impairment make intervention even more likely and the need for early identification and treatment is essential.
2. The patient requires invasive monitoring of blood pressure and CVP, urine output and frequent blood-gas analysis as a

minimum, along with continuous ECG and oxygen saturation monitoring.

(a) Invasive arterial blood pressure monitoring is warranted whenever there is cardiovascular instability when there is the potential for large fluid shifts, or when frequent arterial blood-gas analysis is required. It allows beat-to-beat changes in arterial pressure to be monitored and enables rapid identification of trends or sudden changes in blood pressure; the response to therapeutic measures can be assessed.

(b) CVP (taken as the pressure of blood in the vena cava at the junction with the right atrium) is useful in assessing venous return, intravascular blood volume and right ventricular function. The access can also be used for irritant drug administration dialysis and parenteral nutrition. The CVP varies with respiration in the range 0 to $+8\,cmH_2O$ with inspiration and expiration respectively. More important than any single reading are serial measurements allowing the trend to be followed.

(c) Urine output reflects renal function and general tissue perfusion. An hourly urine output of 0.5–1.0 ml/kg is deemed adequate, although the quality of the urine produced may need to be investigated.

(d) Arterial blood-gas analysis allows insight into the adequacy of respiratory function and/or mechanical ventilation, and also the metabolic state of the patient in terms of acid–base balance.

(e) Gastric tonometry is performed using a modified nasogastric tube which has a distal balloon which may be filled and emptied of fluid. Distilled water is used to fill the balloon when in the stomach, and is allowed to equilibrate with any carbon dioxide there. The distilled water is aspirated and run through a blood-gas analyser. The result, along with that of an arterial blood sample taken at the same time, is used to calculate the intramucosal pH, which correlates closely with the mortality rate. It is a reflection of the adequacy of splanchnic perfusion and a very low gastric intramucosal pH can indicate the presence of gut ischaemia associated with bacteraemia and septicaemia.

The therapy at present for attempting to correct splanchnic underperfusion is with the dopamine receptor agonist dopexamine.

3. (a) *Intra-arterial blood pressure monitoring:* Several sites are suitable for cannulation, although the radial artery is most frequently used because of ease of access. Other sites that may be used include ulnar, brachial, axillary, femoral and the dorsalis pedis artery. Complications associated with cannulation are similar for each site:
  (i)   Arterial thrombosis leading to ischaemia of the area supplied.
  (ii) Infection.
  (iii) Arteriovenous fistula formation.
  (iv) Aneurysm formation.
  (v)   Air embolism.
  (vi) Haemorrhage.
  (b) *Central venous pressure monitoring:* Venous cannulation of a large central vein may be performed at any one of several sites. Each has certain advantages and disadvantages:
  (i)   Internal jugular veins: reliable placement but uncomfortable for the patient.
  (ii) Subclavian veins: less reliable than the internal jugular but more convenient and comfortable for the patient.
  (iii) External jugular veins: easy to perform but it may be difficult to thread the cannula into the subclavian vein to obtain the correct reading.
  (iv) Femoral veins: a long catheter can be used; this is relatively safe and easy to place. Intra-abdominal pathology and obesity will affect the readings and there may be an increased incidence of infection.
  (v)   Arm vein: there is little risk of serious complication but the catheter is often difficult to thread and there is only a 50% chance of it passing into the superior vena cava.

Numerous complications may arise depending on the site chosen:
  (i)   Arterial puncture (difficult to control with subclavian line), haematoma.
  (ii) Arteriovenous fistula.
  (iii) Air embolism.
  (iv) Pneumothorax.
  (v)   Chylothorax.
  (vi) Nerve damage – phrenic, brachial plexus.
  (vii) Subarachnoid puncture.

(viii) Oesophageal puncture.

(ix) Tracheal puncture.

(x) Local/systemic infection.

(xi) Arrhythmias (if the guidewire or catheter enters the right ventricle).

4. The right internal jugular vein is the site most commonly used for CVP in surgical patients as this is the most accessible site for the anaesthetist.

The patient is placed in the Trendelenburg position with the head tilted to the left. With the vein thus distended it is often possible to ballotte the vein in the neck, but if this is not possible then by entering lateral to the carotid artery at the junction of the two hands of sternomastoid and aiming toward the ipsilateral nipple, the vein can usually be entered. The Seldinger technique involves placing a flexible wire through the needle used to locate the vein. The needle is then removed leaving the wire in place, and a dilator fed over the wire. The dilator is then removed, the catheter threaded over the wire and the wire then removed. The catheter is sutured in place, the channels aspirated and flushed, and its position confirmed by chest X-ray.

5. When inotropic agents are required a balloon-tipped flow-directed pulmonary artery catheter (Swan–Ganz catheter) should be inserted. This allows monitoring of left ventricular function and the systemic circulation and the effect of inotropic intervention.

6. The pulmonary artery catheter is placed via central venous access. Its distal lumen is attached to a pressure transducer, and the pressure displayed as a waveform on a screen. On initial introduction of the catheter a CVP tracing will be obtained. The balloon is then inflated. The catheter is advanced and as the tip passes through the tricuspid valve the pressure wave alters to that of a right ventricular trace. Further catheter advancement results in its passage through the pulmonary valve, when the diastolic pressure will increase while the systolic pressure remains the same. Finally the tip of the catheter will pass into one of the small vessels and the balloon will occlude blood flow. The pressure trace will then reflect left atrial pressure and thus left ventricular end-diastolic pressure. The balloon should be deflated to ensure a return to the normal pulmonary artery tracing and only reinflated when a measurement of the wedge pressure (i.e. left atrial pressure) is required.

Both direct and derived parameters can be obtained:
(a) Direct
  (i) CVP: 0–8 mmHg.
  (ii) Right arterial pressure: 0–8 mmHg.
  (iii) Right ventricular pressure: 25/0–8 mmHg.
  (iv) Pulmonary artery pressure: 25/8–12 mmHg.
  (v) Pulmonary artery wedge pressure: 8–12 mmHg.
  (vi) Mixed venous saturation: 85%.
  (vii) Central temperature.
(b) Derived parameters
  (i) Cardiac output: 5 l/min.
  (ii) Cardiac index: 2.8–3.6 l/min per m.
  (iii) Systemic vascular resistance: 770–1500 dyn/s per cm^5.
  (iv) Pulmonary vascular resistance: 20–120 dyn/s per cm^5.
  (v) Oxygen delivery: 600 ml/min per m^2.
  (vi) Oxygen consumption: 150 ml/min per m^2.

Cardiac output is measured by a thermodilution technique. A known volume, usually 10 ml, of cold 5% glucose is rapidly injected through the proximal port and the temperature change at the distal thermistor measured. The cardiac output is automatically calculated from the area under the temperature/time curve obtained.

Complications of the pulmonary artery catheter are those associated with placement of a central venous cannula and in addition:
(a) Venticular rupture.
(b) Valvular damage.
(c) Pulmonary artery rupture.
(d) Thrombosis or infection.
(e) Bundle-branch block.
(f) Ventricular arrhythmias.
(g) Kinking of the catheter.

Mark Smith
Alastair Skelly

Case 13   Chronic pancreatitis

A 45-year-old man presented to the outpatient clinic with a 4-month history of epigastric pain associated with epigastric fullness, diarrhoea and weight loss. Computed tomographic (CT) scan showed calcification in the pancreatic head and a 7 cm cystic lesion in the tail of the pancreas.

Questions

1. What is the likely diagnosis? How would you evaluate this patient?
2. Classify chronic pancreatitis.
3. Discuss management of pain and the indications for surgery in chronic pancreatitis.
4. What is a pseudocyst? How would you classify pseudocysts? What are the complications of pancreatic pseudocyst?

Answers

1. Chronic pancreatitis. Evaluation of a patient with chronic pancreatitis includes assessment of pancreatic structure and exocrine and endocrine function. Ultrasound should be performed to exclude the presence of gallstones, but pancreatic anatomy and the presence of pancreatic calcification are best determined by CT scanning. Visualization of ductal anatomy with endoscopic retrograde cholangiopancreatography (ERCP) is essential when planning drainage or resectional procedures for chronic pancreatitis or pseudocyst. Operation for pseudocyst should be performed soon after ERCP to avoid septic complications. If ERCP is not technically possible then on-table pancreatography can provide the information necessary to make rational intraoperative decisions. Some surgeons routinely perform mesenteric angiography to identify pseudoaneurysm or portal hypertension due to portal or splenic vein thrombosis, the presence of which may influence the management plan.

Assessment of pancreatic function is equally important. Clinical expression of pancreatic functional insufficiency implies that a gross degree of parenchymal destruction (or obstruction) has occurred. It has been estimated that 90% of exocrine secretory capacity must be lost before steatorrhoea occurs. Exocrine function can be measured noninvasively using a fluorescein dilaurate (Pancreolauryl) test which has a sensitivity and specificity in excess of 90%. Endocrine function can be assessed with a standard oral glucose tolerance test.

Formal nutritional assessment is important, as is psychological evaluation, particularly in current or reformed alcohol abusers.

2. Based on the underlying pathogenesis, chronic pancreatitis may be classified into two main types: chronic calcifying (CCP) and obstructive pancreatitis. CCP accounts for 95% of all cases of chronic pancreatitis. CCP represents a similar end-organ response to a variety of different aetiological agents, including alcohol, hypercalcaemia, pancreatic stone protein deficiency in familial chronic pancreatitis and tropical pancreatitis. A causative agent is not identifiable in many cases of CCP. The pathological lesions in CCP are patchily distributed throughout the pancreas. Current evidence suggests that the underlying mechanism involves deposition of proteinaceous plugs within the tubules which form a matrix for calcium deposition, forming calculi.

Obstructive pancreatitis results from occlusion of the pancreatic duct by tumour, congenital anomaly or by stricture persisting after an episode of acute inflammation. This last circumstance provides a mechanism by which choledocholithiasis may lead to the development of chronic pancreatitis, although this situation is probably very rare. In contrast to CCP, the chronic inflammatory lesions in obstructive pancreatitis are uniformly distributed throughout the pancreas.

3. Rational and effective management of chronic pancreatitis requires full evaluation of pancreatic structure and function. Pain is the dominant symptom in patients with chronic pancreatitis. Mild pain may be controlled with non-opiate analgesics. Malnutrition due to pancreatic exocrine insufficiency should be corrected by enzyme supplementation. Functional suppression of pancreatic exocrine secretion using pancreatic enzyme supplements has been suggested

as a potential therapy for pain due to chronic pancreatitis; however, a randomized trial failed to show benefit from this therapy. The principal indications for surgical intervention are chronic pain requiring narcotic analgesics, weight loss, inability to work because of pain and the occurrence of complications of chronic pancreatitis. The choice of procedure should be individualized to suit the patient's situation. Surgical correction of complications of chronic pancreatitis such as pseudocyst or obstruction of the duodenum or bile duct may be effective in relieving pain. Successful management of symptomatic pseudocysts necessitates imaging of the pancreatic duct, by either ERCP or on-table pancreatography. If there is no communication with the pancreatic duct then percutaneous catheter drainage (rather than aspiration) is worth attempting. However, if there is communication with or obstruction of the pancreatic duct then an operative approach is more appropriate. Most chronic pseudocysts can be managed by internal drainage, preferably into a Roux-en-Y jejunal loop. Indications for pancreatic resection for treatment of pseudocyst include discontinuity of the main pancreatic duct, multiple cysts, replacement of a large portion of the pancreas by the pseudocyst and associated pseudoaneurysm formation.

Longitudinal pancreaticojejunostomy reduces pain in 75% of patients with obvious pancreatic duct distension. Surgical repair of common bile duct stricture is indicated even if the patient is asymptomatic if liver function tests are persistently abnormal. In the absence of any of these conditions a number of alternative procedures may be attempted before recommending a resectional procedure to the patient. Coeliac plexus block may produce significant pain reduction in 50% of patients. Thoracoscopic splanchnicectomy is a newer technique that may be effective in relieving pain caused by chronic pancreatitis. The greater and lesser splanchnic nerves are divided through a left thoracoscopic approach, along with the anterior and posterior vagal trunks. Further experience with this technique is required to establish its long-term efficacy in management of pain due to chronic pancreatitis. Open coeliac neurectomy and pancreatic autotransplantation are two alternative pain-relieving procedures that have been advocated, although neither procedure has been widely adopted. Pancreatic resection should only be considered for patients who continue to have disabling pain despite the measures outlined above. The extent of resection is determined by the distribution of the inflammatory changes in the gland and by the functional status of the pancreas, avoiding total pancreatectomy if possible in the patient who is not yet diabetic. When disease is limited mainly to the body and tail of the pancreas, distal pancreatectomy (preserving the spleen where possible) is likely to achieve satisfactory control of pain in more than 80% of patients. Resection of the pancreatic head may be performed as a classical Whipple's resection or with preservation of the pylorus. Resection of the pancreatic head with preservation of the entire duodenum is another option, although this has not gained widespread application because of concern over late development of duodenal stenosis, which occurs in 5–10% of patients.

Close follow-up is mandatory for all patients to detect postoperative exocrine and endocrine failure. Management of endocrine failure may be particularly difficult in these patients due to lack of compensatory glucagon secretion and poor patient compliance with treatment.

4. A pseudocyst is a fluid collection arising in or near the pancreas which has no epithelial lining. The possibility of a cystic neoplasm of the pancreas should always be excluded when dealing with a suspected pseudocyst. Pseudocysts may be classified according to whether they occur following acute or chronic pancreatitis or trauma.

Pseudocysts that follow an episode of acute pancreatitis rarely communicate with the pancreatic duct and are usually extrapancreatic, most commonly in the lesser sac. If possible, they should be treated conservatively for at least 4–6 weeks since many will resolve spontaneously within that time. In addition, internal drainage before 6 weeks is likely to be technically difficult since the wall of the pseudocyst is not 'mature' and will not hold sutures adequately. If treatment is required before this time, percutaneous or external operative drainage is a better option. Size is also an important determinant of the need for intervention. Pseudocysts less than 6 cm in diameter are more likely to resolve spontaneously without complication compared to larger pseudocysts.

In contrast, pseudocysts that occur in association with chronic pancreatitis are usually intrapancreatic surrounded by a rim of pancreatic tissue, associated with abnormalities of the pancreatic duct, and are more likely to communicate with the pancreatic duct. A number of studies have shown that these pseudocysts are unlikely to resolve spontaneously and may be associated with significant morbidity and mortality if treated expectantly.

Traumatic pseudocysts occur as a result of direct injury to the pancreatic ductal system. In most instances the diagnosis of pancreatic ductal injury is delayed. The site of the ductal injury determines the optimum management. Pseudocyst associated with injury to a peripheral duct can be observed since spontaneous resolution may occur. Pseudocyst associated with injury to the distal main pancreatic duct may be treated percutaneously by catheter drainage with reasonable expectation of success. In contrast, pseudocyst resulting from proximal pancreatic duct injury is more likely to require operative management, by internal drainage if the duct communicates with the pseudocyst but is otherwise intact, or by pancreatic resection if the main pancreatic duct is strictured.

The main complications of pseudocysts include infection, local compression, rupture and bleeding. Infection may occur secondary to direct extension from adjacent infected pancreatic tissue or following attempted percutaneous drainage. Pancreatic pseudocysts may also cause compression or obstruction of the stomach, duodenum or common bile duct. Rupture of a pseudocyst may occur into the peritoneal cavity causing peritonitis or pancreatic ascites, into the pleural space causing a pancreaticopleural fistula or into the bowel lumen. The most dramatic complication of pseudocyst is bleeding. Portal or splenic vein thrombosis may lead to portal hypertension with development of oesophageal varices (which, in fact, rarely bleed spontaneously). Pseudoaneurysm of the splenic or gastroduodenal artery is a more frequent cause of bleeding. Angiographic embolization is the first-choice treatment; however, if the patient is haemodynamically unstable then laparotomy with suture ligation of the vessel accompanied by pseudocyst drainage or pancreatic resection is the appropriate treatment.

Further reading

Beger HG, Büchler M, Ditschuneit H and Malfertheiner P. (eds) (1990) *Chronic Pancreatitis.* Springer-Verlag, Heidelberg

Grace PA and Williamson RCN. (1993) Modern management of pancreatic pseudocysts. *British Journal of Surgery* **80**: 573–581

Johnson CD and Imrie CW. (eds) (1991) *Pancreatic Disease. Progress and Prospects.* Springer-Verlag, Heidelberg

Justin Geoghegan
Patrick Broe

Case 14 Small-bowel fistula

A 35-year-old man presented to his general practitioner complaining of general malaise, weight loss, abdominal pain and a purulent discharge from an old abdominal scar. The discharge originated from what was initially a tender red swelling in the wound. The other symptoms were gradual in onset but progressive. Abdominal examination revealed a tender mass in the right iliac fossa and there was a 1 cm defect at the lower end of a right paramedian scar. This was surrounded by a small amount of granulation tissue and there was a bead of pus arising from the hole. He gave a history that, at the age of 19, he had undergone a right hemicolectomy for Crohn's disease.

Questions

1. What is the likely cause for the mass and the discharge?
2. What are the other common causes of this complication?
3. How would you confirm the diagnosis and what other tests might be useful?
4. What are the principles behind the treatment of this complication?

Answers

1. The most likely cause of this patient's problem is a recurrence of Crohn's disease with an inflammatory mass and the development of an enterocutaneous fistula. A less likely cause might be the development of a malignancy. From the history it seems that this man developed an abscess beneath the wound before fistulation.
2. Intestinal fistulas most commonly arise following the breakdown of an anastomosis. The breakdown occurs because of the presence of one or more risk factors, including ischaemia of the bowel ends, tension, distal obstruction, malnutrition, sepsis and involvement of the bowel wall by diseases such as malignancy, radiation enteritis and inflammatory bowel disease.

Inflammatory bowel disease is a common cause of spontaneous fistula formation. Crohn's disease, diverticular disease and tuberculosis are the main diagnoses in this group. Fistulas caused by Crohn's disease can be classified into type 1 (spontaneous formation due to transmural inflammation and penetration by fissuring ulcers) and type 2 (following surgery as a result of anastomotic leakage).

Tuberculosis can often closely mimic Crohn's disease, the true diagnosis being revealed by histology and culture of the tubercle bacillus. Diverticular disease usually causes fistulas by spontaneous drainage of pericolic abscesses. They are most often colovesical or colocutaneous.

Radiotherapy, particularly of the pelvis, gives rise to enteric fistulas which are resistant to treatment.

Malignant disease is another cause of fistula formation resulting from direct invasion of other structures or following surgery. Surgery for malignant fistulas is usually only palliative but may be worthwhile for symptom control.

Trauma is an uncommon cause of fistula formation and may be due to a penetrating injury, sometimes inadvertently caused during a surgical procedure. Rarely fistulas may arise from an ingested foreign body.

3. The diagnosis of the fistula in the above patient was confirmed by performing fistulography. A balloon catheter was gently inserted in to the defect and contrast was instilled. The contrast passed along a narrow track before outlining the neoterminal ileum. Other useful imaging techniques might include a small-bowel enema, a double-contrast barium enema, ultrasound and computed tomography. Useful information can be obtained from the following blood tests: full blood count, urea and electrolytes, arterial blood gases, serum albumin, erythrocyte sedimentation rate, C-reactive protein, zinc and magnesium levels and clotting studies. These blood tests will reveal abnormalities relevant to patients with intestinal fistulas, such as anaemia, evidence of continuing sepsis, evidence of continuing disease activity, electrolyte imbalance, acid–base imbalance and trace element deficiency. In addition to these investigations it is sometimes helpful to perform an endoscopic procedure such as gastroscopy, colonoscopy, cystoscopy and, in the case of pancreatic fistulas, endoscopic retrograde cholangiopancreatography.

4. The principles behind the management of patients with an intestinal fistula follow several phases:

(a) *Resuscitation:* Patients with intestinal fistulas may become dehydrated and when they present are usually suffering from varying degrees of sepsis. The loss of large volumes of electrolyte-rich secretions from high-output fistulas results in metabolic and electrolyte disturbance. Any loss in excess of 500 ml over 24 h is regarded as high output. Fluid and electrolyte replacement should start immediately. It is important to measure all inputs and outputs in order to achieve optimum fluid balance. Reduction of fluid loss can be achieved by the use of proton pump inhibitors or H_2-receptor antagonists, somatostatin and antidiarrhoeal drugs.

(b) *Skin protection:* The secretions from enteric fistulas contain proteolytic enzymes which will rapidly digest skin if they are allowed to come into contact. Stoma bags which drain into a separate reservoir are most efficient. Some fistulas are not suitable for bag collection and may require suction applied through a sump drain device in order to protect the skin. Collection of the effluent allows accurate measurement of the volume and, if necessary, the electrolyte content. The skin around the fistula can be protected by Stomadhesive sheets.

(c) *Control of sepsis:* Sepsis is a major cause of morbidity and mortality in these patients and should be treated aggressively. Abscesses should be suspected if there is pain, pyrexia, leukocytosis and a tachycardia. Once detected they should be drained; this can often be achieved by percutaneous means. A subtle way of detecting hidden sepsis is by performing an indium 111-labelled white-cell scan. When there has been extensive intra-abdominal sepsis or when minimal-access techniques are technically impossible, it is necessary to open up pockets of pus and institute open drainage. Antibiotics are indicated for spreading cellulitis, septicaemia and infection in a normally sterile compartment such as the urinary tract or lower respiratory tract. They should be as specific as possible and not given over prolonged periods of time to prevent the development of resistant bacterial and fungal infections.

(d) *Nutrition:* There is often inadequate functioning bowel available for fluid absorption and food digestion. However, some fistulas arising from the distal small bowel or colon do not interfere significantly with digestion and normal feeding may be satisfactory. All high-output fistulas and those which bypass large segments of bowel will result in rapid dehydration, loss of electrolytes and failure to absorb sufficient nutrients, vitamins and trace elements. It is therefore important to institute nutritional treatment as soon as possible. Enteral feeding is preferable and can be delivered via fine-bore feeding tubes, gastrostomy tubes or jejunostomy tubes. If the small bowel is not available for use or is inadequate, then parenteral nutrition is required. This can be initiated through a peripheral venous line until definitive access is obtained. A tunnelled central venous line provides the most reliable access and modern silicone rubber catheters placed via the cephalic vein into the superior vena cava can last many years if required. All fluid, electrolyte and nutrients can be conveniently contained in a single 'big bag' and infused overnight, leaving the patient free to mobilize during the day.

(e) *Anatomy:* It is a necessity, early on in the management of a fistula, to define its anatomy. The anatomy can be determined by employing the imaging techniques mentioned in the answer to question 3. Endoscopy also plays a part in confirming both the presence of disease and the anatomy of those organs which are accessible.

(f) *Conservative management:* Around 60% of external fistulas will close spontaneously, especially if sepsis has been eliminated, but there are situations where fistulas will not close. Those situations are total separation of the bowel ends, distal obstruction, continuing sepsis and abscess formation around the fistula and mucocutaneous continuity. In addition fistulas are unlikely to close when they arise from a segment of diseased bowel, such as an area of Crohn's disease, or when there is a malignant process occurring. All of the previous principles of treatment such as drainage of sepsis still apply. If there are bad prognostic signs for fistula closure then surgery may be required.

(g) *Surgical treatment:* If, after 6 weeks of conservative treatment, a fistula has not closed, surgical treatment needs to be considered. Before surgery is performed it is imperative if possible that all sepsis has resolved and malnutrition has been corrected. Ideally the serum albumin should be in the normal range. The timing of surgery should be delayed for a minimum of 6 weeks and up to 6 months to allow optimum resolution of inflammation, making surgery technically easier and safer. The incision should be planned to give the widest possible exposure of the abdominal contents. If possible, the incision should be away from previous scars to allow access to the peritoneal cavity. The bowel should be mobilized from the duodenum to the terminal ileum. The fistula and any associated diseased bowel should be resected, leaving healthy tension-free ends with a good blood supply. The bowel should be re-anastomosed and any defect in a healthy viscus should be closed by direct suture. If there is doubt about the viability of the ends of bowel for anastomosis or there is an associated abscess cavity, then they should be exteriorized and closed at a later date. Tenuous anastomoses benefit from the added protection of a temporary loop jejunostomy or ileostomy. Intravenous nutrition should be continued until enteral feeding has become established. Local surgery to a fistula and modification of technique in order to achieve a better cosmetic result usually result in failure.

Further reading

Alexander-Williams J and Irving MH. (1982) *Intestinal Fistulas*. John Wright, Bristol

D.M. Richards
Miles Irving

Case 15 Tracheostomy

A 55-year-old man presented to ENT outpatients with inspiratory stridor, hoarseness and painful swallowing. Examination revealed swelling and fixation of the left hemilarynx leading to airway compromise. A 4 cm node was also palpable in the mid deep cervical chain, from which fine-needle aspiration confirmed the presence of metastatic squamous cell carcinoma. Computed tomography scanning revealed tumour within the larynx with destruction of the thyroid cartilage. Having been staged as a $T_4N_2M_0$ tumour, the patient underwent local anaesthetic tracheostomy to secure the airway, followed by direct laryngoscopic assessment and frozen-section biopsy of the tumour. He was then treated by laryngectomy followed by a 6-week course of radiotherapy.

Questions

1. List the main indications for tracheostomy in both children and adults.
2. What are the essential differences between paediatric and adult tracheostomy?
3. Describe the early complications and their management.
4. What precautions are required with tube cuff care?
5. When should the primary tube be changed?
6. How does the replacement tube differ from the primary tube and how is the former managed?

Answers

1. The main causes for tracheostomy are given in Table 15.1.
2. The indications and anatomical differences between the adult and child make the operation of paediatric tracheostomy very different from its adult counterpart. The main points to appreciate are first, that cuffed tubes are not used in children because the relatively small tracheal diameter does not allow space for a tube of adequate calibre in addition to a cuff. Second, the short neck and a high brachiocephalic vein can cause a low-placed tracheostomy tube to erode into a high brachiocephalic vein with obvious

Table 15.1 Indications for tracheostomy in children and adults

Children
Congenital
  Laryngotracheomalacia
  Bilateral vocal cord palsy
  Laryngeal webs and stenosis
  Subglottic haemangioma
  Laryngeal cysts (cf. cystic hygromas)
  Craniofacial anomalies (e.g. Crouzon's)
  Syndromes (Treacher Collins, Pierre Robin)

Acquired
  Laryngeal papillomatosis
  Tumours, e.g. rhabdomyosarcoma
  Infection (cf. epiglottitis)

Adults
Neoplastic
  Malignant – squamous cell carcinoma, sarcomas, etc.
  Benign (rare) – chondromas, pleomorphic adenoma, lipoma, fibroma

Autoimmune
  Sarcoid
  Wegener's granulomatosis

Infective
  Diphtheria
  Tuberculosis
  Syphilis

Traumatic
  Laryngeal trauma from blunt or penetrating injuries
  Iatrogenic from thyroid, neck and chest surgery

Respiratory
  Chronic obstructive airway disease (rare)
  Obstructive sleep apnoea
  Long-term ventilation

Neurological
  Bilateral vocal cord palsy *but never* for treatment of aspiration

consequences. If this is technically unavoidable, the vein should be protected by a muscle flap. Third, the opening into the paediatric trachea must be made by a vertical slit and *never* by removing cartilage. This is because the relatively smaller tracheal diameter makes stenosis more likely to occur following decannulation, and almost all children have their tube ultimately removed. Finally, the inferiorly based tracheal flap of Björk, although still used in both children and adults, should not be used in either as it is potentially dangerous and offers few – if any – benefits. Because of tension and dynamic movement of the trachea upon swallowing and breathing, the flap often becomes separated from its cutaneous attachment. It can easily prolapse or be pushed back into the trachea during a tube change, leading to loss of the airway.

3. Tracheostomy in general should be a straightforward operation provided good surgical principles are adhered to and the tissues are handled with respect. With relevance to the latter issue, use of bipolar diathermy should be encouraged. Despite these considerations tracheostomy has many potential complications, ranging from minor to lethal. Early complications are confined to those that arise from damage to regional anatomical structures, such as recurrent nerves, pleural reflections, great vessels, thyroid, oesophagus. The common complications include bleeding from the anterior jugular veins or thyroid, tube displacement, surgical emphysema and wound infection. Complications are minimized by performing dissection in a controlled manner through tissue planes and identifying relevant structures. Dissection should always be in the midline and the thyroid isthmus should always be divided and transfixed to allow precise identification of the tracheal rings so that the tracheostomy can be placed between the second and fifth rings. Once absolute haemostasis has been achieved, the tracheostomy is made as a vertical slit. This must not be made too long, otherwise this will predispose to air leaks around the tube and surgical emphysema. Postoperatively bleeding around the tube may be controlled by Surgicel and cottonoids soaked in topical adrenaline to effect tamponade, particularly if it is low-pressure venous bleeding. Brisk arterial bleeds may require return to theatre. Surgical emphysema may be controlled by reopening the wound, thereby creating a line of least resistance for air escape. The cuff should also be checked to ensure that it has been sufficiently inflated. The patient should be placed on a broad-spectrum antibiotic and this settles in 2–3 days. Tube displacement should be avoided by either stitching the tube to the skin or securing it with double tapes so that the tape tension on each side may be adjusted appropriately. The correct tension should allow one finger in the child and two in the adult to pass underneath the tapes from the back of the neck when the head is flexed at the shoulders.

Great care must be taken when replacing a displaced tube so that false passages are not created. It is not always obvious that the tube has been correctly placed, even if air flow and ventilation appear correct. When a displaced tube is replaced it is wise to pass a nasendoscope, to be fully sure of tube position. Damage to the anterior wall of the oesophagus, if not recognized immediately at the time of surgery, should be treated conservatively by nasogastric feeding for 7–10 days and antibiotics.

4. Care of the tube and cuff are of paramount importance. As the nose is bypassed by tracheostomy, inspired air is no longer warmed, filtered and humidified. All tracheostomy patients, therefore, require humidification of air for the first few days until the lower airway adapts to this radical physiological change. Because cough is impaired, regular suction by sterile catheters is also necessary. Only high-volume low-pressure cuffs should be used. Ideally cuff pressures should be checked by a commercial manometer to ensure that pressure is not above capillary perfusion pressure. If not available, the cuff should be deflated for 5 min each hour. High cuff pressures greater than capillary perfusion will induce mucosal necrosis which will be circumferential, leading to tracheal stenosis some months later once the scar tissue is established and mature.

5. The cuffed tracheostomy tube should be changed to a cuffless tube once all bleeding around the wound has stopped and a track has established itself. This will require a minimum of 5 days and the optimal time for tube change should be at 1 week.

6. In the adult or older child the replacement tube, unlike the primary cuffed tube, may consist of four parts. These are an outer and inner tube, obturator and valved inner tube to promote speech. The inner tube is always slightly longer than the outer tube, so that crusting of the latter will never lead to a situation where the airway is compromised. The outer tube can be left *in situ* long-term but the inner tube requires regular removal and cleaning. The frequency of cleaning, however, is empirical but should be at least once daily. The obturator facilitates replacement of the outer tube when this is removed for cleaning. The valved inner tube allows inspiration through the tracheostomy but expired air passes around the tube and through the larynx in the usual manner, thereby permitting speech. At night the speaking

valve should be changed to the non-valved inner tube for obvious reasons. After a week humidification of inspired air should no longer be necessary but a muffler is advisable to prevent large particulate matter entering the tracheostomy tube.

Further reading

Rogers JH. (1987) Tracheostomy and decannulation. In: Evans JNG (ed.) *Scott-Brown's Otolaryngology*, 5th edn. *Paediatric Otolaryngology.* Butterworths, Oxford

Neil S. Tolley

Case 16 Regional anaesthesia

A 65-year-old man is admitted for a revision of a left total hip replacement. The first operation was performed 7 years previously after he had fallen off a ladder while drunk and fractured the neck of his femur, which subsequently became necrotic. Although initially successful, he is now unable to walk because of the pain.

His past medical history includes severe long-standing respiratory disease secondary to smoking which leaves him breathless on minimal exertion.

A year ago he underwent a transurethral resection of the prostate (TURP) under spinal anaesthesia, which was uneventful, but now he complains that his urinary symptoms are beginning to return.

He is still drinking up to half a bottle of spirits a day and continues to smoke between 20 and 40 cigarettes a day.

The anaesthetist decides to perform an epidural block and keep the patient breathing spontaneously with only very light sedation.

Questions

1. What is the difference between an epidural and a spinal block?
2. (a) What are the absolute and relative contraindications to a regional technique?
   (b) What tests would be relevant in this patient?
3. What are the advantages of an epidural block in this patient over (a) a general anaesthetic and (b) spinal block, which he had successfully had for the last operation?
4. List the complications of an epidural block.

Answers

1. The principal difference between an epidural and a spinal block is the site of placement of the drug to be used (usually a local anaesthetic or opioid). For a spinal block the dural and arachnoid meninges are breached and the drug injected directly into the subarachnoid space. Technically

this is done below the level of the termination of the spinal cord (L2/3 in adults, L3/4 in the term neonate and somewhere in between in children).

2. (a) The *absolute* contraindications to regional block are:
   (i) Patient refusal.
   (ii) Any condition predisposing to bleeding – coagulopathies, low platelets, etc.
   (iii) Local sepsis around the proposed puncture site.
   (iv) Lack of experience in the technique.

   Relative contraindications include:
   (i) Heart disease leading to a fixed cardiac output (so that the patient is unable to cope with sympathetic block and hypotension).
   (ii) Hypovolaemia (bleeding and dehydration).
   (iii) Generalized infection or sepsis.

   (b) As this man is a heavy drinker, he may well have liver disease, so a clotting screen should be done to ensure a normal prothrombin time.

   (If he is prescribed subcutaneous heparin, this should be given after the epidural catheter has been inserted, to minimize the chance of an extradural haematoma developing.)

   An ECG and chest X-ray should be performed. These may, however, be normal in the presence of severe ischaemic heart disease or alcohol-induced cardiomyopathy.

3. (a) The advantages of an epidural block over general anaesthesia are that his airway and breathing are not compromised – the epidural block will not compromise his respiratory muscles or depress his ventilation as a general anaesthetic would. He will not require intubation, which may induce bronchospasm and coughing, especially at the end of the operation.

   The epidural block, once instituted, provides a steady haemodynamic state in which there are no major fluctuations in blood pressure. In general, the blood pressure can be maintained on the low side in order to minimize intraoperative blood loss. (In addition, unopposed parasympathetic activity causes the gut to contract down, which aids intra-abdominal surgery.)

   (b) The advantages of an epidural block over spinal anaesthesia are that a spinal block is used as a one-shot technique with a fixed dose of anaesthetic. One of the side-effects is hypotension, which can be difficult to control. With an epidural catheter, the block can be instituted gradually and smoothly, with no rapid or pronounced haemodynamic changes which may strain a potentially damaged heart. The catheter can be used to top-up the block should the operation take longer than 1 h.

4. *Immediate complications*
   (a) Dural puncture – free flow of cerebrospinal fluid through the epidural needle or catheter. This in itself is not serious as it is intentional in a spinal. The Tuohy needle, however, is of 16 or 18 gauge and makes a relatively large hole, through which cerebrospinal fluid may leak for some time, leading to a low-pressure headache.
   (b) Total spinal block – due to injection of relatively large amounts of local anaesthetic into the subarachnoid, instead of epidural, space. This necessitates immediate resuscitation with intravenous fluids plus a vasopressor, intubation and ventilation until the block wears off. Adequate sedation while waiting is also important.
   (c) Hypotension – this is very common and is due to sympathetic blockade leading to vasodilatation. Treatment is with intravenous fluids and vasopressors such as ephedrine or methoxamine.
   (d) Intravenous injection into the epidural veins. This is possible even if no blood is detected on aspiration of needle or catheter. If only a small amount of local anaesthetic is administered, the block simply will not work. Otherwise, systemic toxicity may follow. This is manifest by perioral numbness, tingling in hands and feet, cardiac depression and arrhythmias, hypotension, respiratory depression, convulsions and coma.
   (e) Local anaesthetic overdose. The maximum recommended doses of local anaesthetics are:
       (i) Bupivacaine 2 mg/kg (5 mg/kg when used with 1 in 200 000 adrenaline).
       (ii) Lignocaine 3 mg/kg (7 mg/kg when used with 1 in 200 000 adrenaline).
   (f) Allergy to local anaesthetic – theoretical, but in practice almost unknown with amide-linked local anaesthetics such as bupivacaine.
   (g) Shivering.
   (h) Pruritus – a complication most likely when opioids are used.

(i) Nausea and vomiting – often the first sign of falling blood pressure.

Later complications

(a) Headache – secondary to dural puncture.

(b) Backache – due to the local trauma of the procedure or to lying in an awkward position on the operating table, exacerbated by the fact that the back muscles are relaxed during the period of block.

Severe backache postoperatively may be the first symptom of a space-occupying lesion (see below).

(c) (i) Incomplete block – unilateral or missed segment.

    (ii) Incomplete block of visceral afferents – nausea when abdominal organs are handled.

(d) Extradural haematoma – this is a neurosurgical emergency because of impending spinal cord compression leading to permanent paraplegia.

(e) Bacteraemia – an extradural abscess may develop with neurological sequelae as above.

(f) Urinary retention – this is relevant in this patient who has symptoms of urinary outflow obstruction, despite a TURP in the past.

(g) Neurological sequelae – paraesthesia, including from positioning on the operating table, Horner's syndrome, cauda equina syndrome, spinal nerve neuropathy due to trauma at insertion and leading to paraesthesia, pain and numbness over the distribution of the affected spinal nerve.

(h) Anterior spinal artery syndrome – a rare sequel to hypotension, resulting in postoperative painless paraplegia with preservation of the posterior columns.

(i) Adhesive arachnoiditis – an irritant injectate may cause various degrees of neurological deficit which is often progressive with pain and paralysis.

Further reading

Aitkenhead AR and Smith G. (1990) *Textbook of Anaesthesia* 2nd edn, chaps 1 and 26. Churchill Livingstone, Edinburgh

Helena Scott
Alastair Skelly

Case 17 The management of enterocutaneous fistulas: the importance of parenteral nutrition

A 65-year-old man was admitted having had a significant haematemesis and melaena. Systolic blood pressure on admission was 90 mmHg with a tachycardia of 120 beats/min. Endoscopy showed a very large posterior duodenal ulcer with an active arterial bleeding point visible in the centre. Attempts at laser coagulation were unsuccessful. The patient continued to bleed and after a 6 unit transfusion he was taken to theatre. An emergency Polya gastrectomy was carried out. His immediate postoperative recovery was uneventful but on the sixth postoperative day he developed a high swinging fever and on the eighth postoperative day he developed a bile-stained leak through a suction drain. The total volume of leakage in the first 24 h was 900 ml.

Questions

1. What is an enterocutaneous fistula? What are the common causes of such development and what is the associated mortality?
2. Describe those factors which mitigate against spontaneous fistula closure.
3. Outline a management plan for patients with high-output enterocutaneous fistulas.
4. What are the indications for total parenteral nutrition?
5. Describe how parenteral nutrition can be administered and outline your reasons for using different techniques.
6. Briefly describe the principles that are important in deciding upon fluid and nutrients required in patients with enterocutaneous fistulas.

Answers

1. An enterocutaneous fistula is defined as an abnormal passage or communication leading from an internal organ,

usually a viscus, to the surface of the body. The word is derived from the Latin *fistula*, meaning pipe or flute, and refers to a long, narrow, suppurating canal connecting normally unrelated structures.

Enterocutaneous fistulas most commonly appear secondary to abdominal surgery. Other causes include inflammatory bowel disease, cancer, radiation and trauma. Rare cases are due to foreign bodies, hernias and unusual infections.

The mortality rate for gastrointestinal fistulas ranges between 6 and 30%. Mortality is doubled when fistula output is >500 ml/24 h and is higher in patients with malignant disease or those with radiation enteritis. There is evidence to suggest that the presence of severe malnutrition also increases mortality.

2. The factors which mitigate against spontaneous fistula closure can be summarized as follows:

(a) Loss of bowel continuity such as occurs following complete disruption of an anastomosis.

(b) Distal obstruction. Anastomotic breakdown in association with distal obstruction guarantees that spontaneous closure of the fistula cannot occur. This situation can occur, for example, in patients who have undergone a right hemicolectomy who have previously unsuspected distal colonic obstruction, possibly from an unrecognized colonic tumour or in patients with Crohn's disease from previously undiagnosed distal strictures. Distal obstruction can occur throughout the small intestine from adhesions.

(c) An adjacent abscess cavity through which the fistula drains will also prevent closure. Treatment of abscesses in association with fistulas is a priority in their management.

(d) Spontaneous closure of a fistula is improbable if there is abnormal tissue at the site of fistulation. For example, underlying inflammatory bowel disease, radiation or malignancy may all predispose to persistent fistula losses. To confirm a diagnosis of malignancy it is sometimes necessary to obtain a biopsy specimen of the mucosa through the fistulous tract.

(e) Epithelialization of the fistulous tract down to the opening into the bowel usually precludes spontaneous closure.

(f) The presence of a foreign body such as a suture or prosthetic material.

3. The management of all enterocutaneous fistulas can be summarized as follows:

   (a) Resuscitation and treatment of sepsis.
   (b) Diagnosis.
   (c) Conservative management and nutritional support.
   (d) Definitive surgical therapy.

   (a) Many patients who develop an enterocutaneous fistula initially present with septicaemia and abdominal pain as the fistula contents discharge through an abdominal incision or drain site. The first priority in the management of these patients is resuscitation with crystalloids, control of circulatory and pulmonary failure and the administration of antibiotics.

   Many fistulas are associated with sepsis both as local abscess formation as well as generalized septicaemia. Treatment of septicaemia with appropriate antibiotics and identification of abscess cavities using ultrasound or computed tomography (CT) is essential before embarking upon subsequent stages of fistula management. Focal collections within the abdomen, around the fistula, under the diaphragm, in the paracolic gutters or in the pelvis require drainage either by ultrasound-guided or CT-guided needle aspiration or, sometimes, surgically. In the event that surgical drainage is necessary it is imperative that no attempt is made to close the fistula surgically. This is invariably associated with a recurrence and carries a high mortality rate. It is appropriate at this stage only to drain abscesses and, if appropriate, to bring out a defunctioning loop of intestine. These temporary procedures are used to control the fistula and permit evolution of management to the next stage.

   (b) Once the patient is stable and sepsis is controlled it is appropriate to investigate the patient to establish the cause of the fistula. These investigations will also be directed to excluding those factors outlined above that decrease the chance of spontaneous closure of a fistula. Investigation of the patient will include X-ray techniques such as fistulography where dye is injected down the fistulous tract in association with small-bowel enemas and barium enemas. Other simple diagnostic modalities which help localize the site of origin of the fistula include injection of diluted methylene blue and biochemical analysis of the fistulous output. Biochemistry enables differentiation between serum, pancreatic, biliary, small-bowel or urinary tract origins of fistulous drainage. A plain film of the abdomen should be taken in all cases to exclude the presence of a radiopaque foreign body. Within this stage of management it is important to establish the nature of the fistulous loss and to exclude abnormal tissue at the site of fistula leakage and it is essential to ensure that distal obstruction does not exist.

(c) Conservative management. This necessitates consideration of three areas of therapy:
   (i) Drainage and skin protection.
   (ii) Pharmacological means of reducing fistula output.
   (iii) Fluid and electrolyte management and nutritional support.

   (i) Drainage and skin protection. Fistula drainage from the small bowel contains activated pancreatic enzymes that are corrosive to the skin. Protection against skin laceration is carried out using a combination of some suction, stoma bags and skin barriers such as Stomadhesive or karaya paste. Excellent nursing care is a prerequisite of fistula management success.

   (ii) The conservative management of patients with enterocutaneous fistulas may last for as little as a few days to many months. The aim of the therapy is to maintain the patient in fluid and electrolyte balance without nutritional depletion until such time as spontaneous fistula closure occurs. Conservative management is discontinued when the patient is stable and a decision is made to undertake definitive surgery or if surgery is considered essential as the patient has one or other condition that dictates that spontaneous closure is unlikely to occur.

   Many pharmaceutical agents have been recommended to reduce fistula output. The use of the somatostatin analogue octeotride is gaining increased support; many studies now attest to its value, particularly in patients with high-output fistulas. The use of nasogastric aspiration is controversial unless patients have confirmed small-bowel obstruction. Further, certain authors have advocated the use of a gastrostomy tube but again this has not gained general acceptance. H_2-receptor antagonists are associated with a decrease in fistula output but probably not when used in conjunction with octreotide.

(iii) Fluid and electrolyte management and nutritional support (see answer 6).

(d) Definitive surgical therapy. Elective surgical therapy is only contemplated when infection is controlled, the patient's nutritional status is satisfactory and conservative measures have failed. The surgical techniques used vary depending upon the anatomical site of the fistula. The duodenal fistulas usually necessitate resection and primary neoanastomosis. A duodenal stump fistula will usually close spontaneously but if necessary can be treated by debridement and an attempt at new closure. Alternatively, it can be converted to a controlled duodenal fistula using a Foley catheter within the duodenal stump. Small-bowel fistulas usually require simple closure, bypass or primary resection. Colonic fistulas which persist are usually as a consequence of distal obstruction which requires appropriate surgical therapy.

4. Total parenteral nutrition is indicated for those patients who have temporary or permanent intestinal failure. Intestinal failure may be defined as that condition which occurs when a patient's intestinal tract is unable to digest and absorb an adequate supply of nutrients. Permanent intestinal failure occurs in patients who have no small intestine and these patients may be candidates for long-term home parenteral nutrition. Temporary intestinal failure may occur as a consequence of disease or medical intervention. Short-term intestinal failure is therefore a common accompaniment following major excisional surgery in patients who have a temporary ileus or in patients with enterocutaneous fistulas. Temporary intestinal failure may also occur because of medical intervention if the attending clinician feels that enteral nutrition should be discontinued as, for example, frequently occurs in the conservative management of patients with inflammatory bowel disease as part of the concept of bowel rest.

5. Parenteral nutrition is traditionally administered through a central venous line. An infraclavicular subclavian cannulation is the most commonly used technique, although parenteral nutrition is frequently given through a cannula inserted into the cephalic vein which is then, under image intensification, fed into the superior vena cava. The tip of a central venous line should lie within the superior vena cava to minimize risks of subclavian venous thrombosis. Central venous cannulation is associated with significant morbidity and, for this reason, many clinicians now advocate the use of peripheral parenteral nutrition. This is appropriate for most surgical patients but not in those with inadequate peripheral veins, those with specific nutritional requirements or those who require very prolonged parenteral nutrition of periods of 2 weeks or more. Further, peripheral parenteral nutrition does limit the flexibility of the prescriber. Peripheral parenteral nutrition necessitates the use of certain regimens which have an osmolality <800 mosmol/l which can be tolerated by peripheral veins for limited periods. Many clinicians now advocate the use of fine-bore infant feeding tubes inserted through a cephalic vein and left *in situ* for as long as possible, whilst others prefer the technique of cyclical infusion of nutrients with rotation of venous access sites.

6. Fluid requirements and nutritional need. It is essential to bear in mind that fluid and electrolyte management is an integral part of the conservative therapy of patients with enterocutaneous fistulas and should be considered alongside their nutritional requirements. Blood is required to maintain haemodynamic stability. Hypoalbuminaemia is common and it is a consequence of sepsis. Hypoalbuminaemia is not an indication for albumin replacement. Parenteral fluid replacement is calculated by adding the fistula output per day +1500 ml for urine output +500 ml for any additional losses such as those from nasogastric aspiration. This determines the total fluid volume required per day, assuming that the patient has a normal renal function. Specific requirements for electrolytes are estimated by sending samples of urine, nasogastric aspirate and fistula output for electrolyte and mineral determinations. Knowledge of a patient's daily volume and electrolyte requirements permits commencement of fluid and electrolyte therapy. A knowledge of gastrointestinal tract secretion provides useful information

Table 17.1 Composition of gastrointestinal secretions

Intestinal tract locality	Volume (ml)	Na (mmol/l)	K (mmol/l)	Cl (mmol/l)	HCO_3^- (mmol/l)
Saliva	1500	10	25	10	30
Gastric juice (fasting)	1500	60	15	90	15
Pancreatic fistula	700	140	5	75	120
Biliary fistula	500	145	5	100	40
Jejunostomy	2–3000	110	5	100	30
Ileostomy	500	115	8	45	30
Proximal colostomy	300	80	20	45	30
Diarrhoeal stools	500–15 000	120	25	90	45

(Table 17.1). Note that the content of intestinal losses varies depending upon the anatomical site of loss.

It is important to consider that the aim of nutritional support is to preserve body composition and minimize further losses of protein and energy stores. It is unrealistic to anticipate significant gains of lean body mass unless parenteral nutrition has been given for many months. Parenteral nutrition comprises the simultaneous administration of protein and energy together with minerals, trace elements, vitamins and electrolytes as determined by the patient's requirements. Protein is now always given as a crystalline amino acid and in the majority of patients 0.2 g N/ kg per day will suffice. Higher requirements are indicated in severely stressed patients but these are usually of short duration. Energy requirement can be measured by indirect calorimetry or assessed from various tables such as those of Harris Benedict, but in practice it is usually sufficient to administer 30–35 kcal/kg per day. Energy should be provided as a combination of glucose as carbohydrate source and an intravenous fat emulsion. Significant morbidity is associated with the over-provision of energy. Few surgical patients will ever require more than 2000 kcal/day. There are many proprietary preparations available for the administration of trace elements and vitamins. A summary of their requirements is shown in Tables 17.2 and 17.3.

Parenteral nutrition should be continued until the patient is able to take adequate amounts of nutrients by the enteral route. It is unwise to discontinue parenteral nutrition precipitously. Careful monitoring of fluid and electrolyte losses,

Table 17.2 Recommended daily allowances of trace elements

Element	Effect of deficiency	Dietary*	Intravenous
Iron	Anaemia	2 mg	2 mg
Zinc‡	Impaired wound healing and growth, dermatitis, alopecia	15 mg	4–10 mg§
Copper	Anaemia, neutropenia, bone demineralization	2–3 mg	0.5 mg†
Chromium	Impaired glucose handling	0.05–0.2 mg	10–15 μg†
Iodine	Goitre, hypothyroidism	150 μg	150 μg
Fluorine	Dental susceptibility to caries	1.5–4 mg	0.4 mg
Manganese	Vitamin K deficiency	2–3 mg	0.15–0.8 mg†
Molybdenum	Neurological abnormalities	100 μg	100–200 μg
Selenium	Muscle weakness and pain	20–50 μg	40–120 μg

* Committee on Dietary Allowances (1980).
† Nutrition Advisory Group (1979).
‡ Excessive losses of zinc are not uncommon in surgical patients and clinical zinc deficiency syndromes were first described in such patients. Patients with diarrhoea or ileostomies lose about 17 mg of zinc per litre of faeces, but for patients with a high small-bowel fistula the losses are proportionately less – about 12 mg/l of fistula discharge.
§ If given as zinc sulphate, this needs to be multiplied by 2.5. As only 20% of orally administered zinc is absorbed, a further multiplication by 5 is required if given orally. Zinc levels in the blood reflect zinc ingestion rather than balance. While 4 mg of elemental zinc is sufficient for parenteral regimens, to maintain most patients in zinc balance many surgical patients require more than this and 10 mg as a base requirement is suggested.

blood glucose, serum triglyceride, phosphate, magnesium and zinc are essential during parenteral nutrition. It should be remembered that most morbidity related to total parenteral nutrition is a consequence of the over-infusion of nutrients.

P.M. Murchan
J. MacFie

Table 17.3 Recommended allowances for vitamins

	Action	Effect of deficiency	Dietary*	Intravenous†
Water-soluble				
Thiamine (B$_1$)	Glucose metabolism	Beriberi	1.4 mg	3 mg/day
Riboflavine (B$_2$)	Energy transfer	Glossitis dermatitis	1.6 mg	3.6 mg/day
Nicotinic acid (niacin) (B$_3$)	Energy transfer	Pellagra	18 mg	40 mg/day
Pyridoxine (B$_6$)	Decarboxylation and transamination	Muscle weakness, seizures	2.2 mg	4 mg/day
Pantothenic acid	Component of CoA	Fatigue, muscle cramps	7 mg	15 mg/day
Folate	Coenzyme with B$_{12}$	Anaemia	400 μg	400 μg/day
B$_{12}$	Coenzyme with nucleic acid synthesis	Pernicious anaemia	3 μg	5 mg/day
C	Collagen synthesis	Scurvy	60 mg	100 mg/day
Fat-soluble				
A	Glycoprotein synthesis	Night blindness	1000 μg RE‡	2500 iu/day
D	Calcium and phosphate utilization	Rickets	5 μg	5 μg/day
E	Energy transfer	Neurological disorder	10 mg§	50 mg§/day
K	Prothrombin synthesis	Bleeding disorder	NR¶	10 mg/week

* Committee on Dietary Allowances (1980) (males 23–50 years old).
† Nutrition Advisory Group (1979).
‡ Retinol equivalents. 1 μg retinol equivalent corresponds to 1 μg retinol or 3.33 iu.
§ Alpha-tocopherol equivalents. 1 mg alpha-tocopherol equivalent has the same activity as 0.67 mg d-alpha-tocopherol.
¶ No recommendation.

Case 18 Scoring systems in major trauma

Early one morning, a 23-year-old man was riding to work on his motorcycle along a fast dual carriageway when a car emerged from a side road without warning. His motorcycle struck the car, and he was thrown into the air, and landed on the central crash barrier, sustaining a severe blow to the right side of his chest and injuries to the right leg. He was taken to the local accident and emergency department where his blood pressure was found to be 125/105 mmHg, Glasgow Coma Scale 15 and respiratory rate 34 breaths/min. He was promptly referred to the surgical registrar, who interpreted a supine chest X-ray as being underpenetrated and showing multiple bilateral rib fractures with no evidence of pneumothorax or haemothorax. Shortly afterwards, the patient's blood pressure fell dramatically and he suffered a cardiac arrest; the cardiac monitor showed electromechanical dissociation. The patient died and at postmortem was found to have six fractured ribs on the right side and three on the left side and a large right-sided haemothorax. A compound fracture of the right tibia and an undisplaced fracture of the right superior pubic ramus were also present.

Questions

1. What were the effects of the patient's injuries and what pitfalls were present?
2. Were any of the patient's physiological findings abnormal? What physiological score relevant to trauma could be calculated from them?
3. What anatomical scoring system could be used to classify the patient's injuries?
4. The surgical registrar is asked to present this case at the morbidity and mortality meeting. What scoring system could be used to determine whether this case was an expected or unexpected death?
5. How is information like this used in national trauma audit in both the UK and USA?

Answers

1. From the history of the injury, where much of the force of the impact was taken on the patient's chest, severe chest injuries would be likely. This patient had multiple right-sided rib fractures, associated with severe haemorrhage into the right side of the chest. It is easy to misinterpret diffuse opacity of a supine/portable chest X-ray as being due to underpenetration – in this case a large amount of blood had collected in the right side of the chest and the asymmetry of the lung fields was a clue to the diffuse haemothorax.

2. The patient's blood pressure, with a narrowed pulse pressure and raised diastolic reading, was indicative of stage II shock (blood loss around 750–1500 ml). The respiratory rate was raised, probably due to the physiological effects of blood loss rather than chest injury.

   The most commonly used physiological scoring system in current practice is the Revised Trauma Score (RTS) (Table 18.1). This score is used in two forms – the triage version makes use of unweighted values derived from the Glasgow Coma Scale (GCS). Systolic blood pressure and respiratory rate are used in the USA by paramedics to decide the need for transport to a trauma centre, and by UK accident and emergency departments in deciding the need for senior advice or a trauma team.

   The full revised trauma score is used in trauma audit. Weighting factors need to be used to adjust the raw coded values for GCS, systolic blood pressure and respiratory rate.

   An example for this patient is shown in Table 18.2.

   The use of this final value in trauma audit is discussed below.

3. The most widely accepted method of assessing injury severity from anatomical information is the Injury Severity Score (ISS), which is calculated by the following method:
   (a) All of the patient's injuries are listed as fully as possible.
   (b) Injuries are sorted into six categories by body region: head or neck; face; chest; abdominal or pelvic contents; extremities or pelvic girdle; external (including burns).
   (c) The Abbreviated Injury Scale (AIS; 1990 revision) is used to score each of the specific injuries. This scale gives a numerical value for each injury ranging between 1 (mild) and 5 (severe, life-threatening). Injuries which are expected to be universally fatal (e.g. decapitation) are

Table 18.1 Revised trauma score

		Coded value		
Systolic blood pressure		>89	4	
(mmHg)		76–89	3	
		50–75	2	→
		1–49	1	
		0	0	_____
Respiratory rate		10–29	4	
(breaths/min)		>29	3	
		6–9	2	→
		1–5	1	
		0	0	_____

Glasgow Coma Scale (GCS)

Eye opening

Spontaneous	4	13–15	4	
To voice	3	9–12	3	
To pain	2	6–8	2	→
None	1	4–5	1	
		3	0	_____

Verbal response

Oriented	5	
Confused	4	If any of these totals
Inapproriate words	3	are less than 4,
Incomprehensible words	2	*inform the senior*
None	1	*doctor on call*

Motor response

Obeys command	6
Localizes	5
Withdraws	4
Abnormal flexion	3
Abnormal extension	2
None	1

Total GCS points _____

Table 18.2 How the revised trauma score is attained

Parameter	Value	Coded value	Weighting factor	Result
Glasgow Coma Score	15	4	0.9368	3.7472
Systolic blood pressure (mmHg)	130	4	0.7326	2.9304
Respiratory rate (breaths/min)	34	3	0.2908	0.8724
Revised trauma score = 7.5452				

listed as having a score of 6, but this score is not used in the calculation of the ISS. AIS 90 has been validated for use in calculating the ISS for trauma audit purposes.

(d) The highest AIS score in each body region, for a maximum of three body regions, and the coded values are squared and added together. An example for this patient is shown in Table 18.3.

Table 18.3

Body region	Injuries	Abbreviated Injury Scale Score	Sum of squares
Chest	6 rib fractures (R) with haemothorax	4	16
	2 rib fractures (L)	2	
Extremities and pelvic girdle	Superior pubic ramus fracture	2	
	Compound tibial fracture (R)	3	9
	Injury Severity Score		25

It can be seen that the maximum ISS would be 75 (three injuries in different regions with an AIS of 5. ISS has been used alone in predicting mortality, but it is non-linear and peaks of deaths occur influenced by single, severe injuries around ISS 16 and 25. The use of ISS in trauma audit is described below.

4. With a knowledge of the revised trauma score and the ISS for a patient, the outcome (death or recovery) can be compared against expected outcome derived from large databases held in both the UK and USA. From these databases, charts have been derived showing a 50% mortality risk line (see below). Four separate charts are necessary, for penetrating and blunt injuries in patients under and over the age of 55 years. The line on these charts resembles the LD_{50} value in clinical pharmacology. The patient's parameters

can be plotted on this chart, and if death occurs at a locus situated below the line, the death is audited as an unexpected outcome. The raised trauma score and ISS of the patient in this case history are plotted in Figure 18.1, and it can be seen that an unexpected death has occurred. For hospitals seeing large numbers of trauma patients, this method is a good way of flagging appropriate cases for discussion at morbidity and mortality meetings – in this example there are clearly educational lessons to be learnt regarding the interpretation of physiological changes and X-ray investigations.

5. As well as undertaking local audit, the hospital can send its results for trauma patient outcome, together with physiological and anatomical details, to the UK Major Trauma Outcome Study (UKMTOS). UKMTOS staff provide confidential comparative feedback to the participant institution, as well as collecting data for the ongoing study.

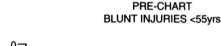

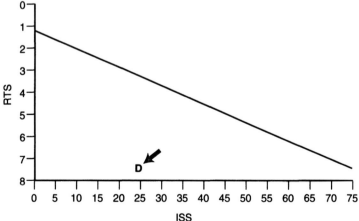

Figure 18.1 Sample pre-chart for blunt trauma patients under the age of 55. The patient in the example is plotted as the letter D.

RTS = Revised trauma score; ISS = Injury Severity Score.

Further reading

Moore EE, Mattox LK and Feliciano DV. (1991) *Trauma*, 2nd edn. Appleton and Lang, Norwalk, CT

Robert Cocks

Case 19 The importance of tissue typing in transplantation

A 49-year-old woman was referred from her local district general hospital for maintenance haemodialysis and consideration for acceptance on to the local renal transplant waiting list. Following the birth of her daughter she had reached end-stage renal failure and received a cadaveric renal transplant in 1991, which failed due to chronic rejection 6 months ago. On screening, the patient's serum contained cytotoxic human leukocyte antigen (HLA) alloantibodies that lysed 80% of a panel of randomly selected third-party cells with a wide diversity of HLA types.

Questions

1. When considering a renal transplant, what are the requirements for matching between donor and recipient?
2. Briefly describe (a) the structure and (b) function of the HLA system.
3. How are the HLA genes inherited and what is linkage disequilibrium?
4. What are the techniques used for prospective HLA matching?
5. How important is matching for HLA in renal transplantation?
6. What are the difficulties associated with the sensitized patient and a positive cross-match result?

Answers

1. Renal transplantation is the treatment of choice for the management of end-stage renal disease in suitable patients. While patient survival is excellent (<5% mortality/year), 10–15% of grafts fail due to acute rejection during the first year and there is a continuing attrition, such that 10-year survival is approximately 50%.

    Three kinds of antigen are carried by allogeneic tissues and stimulate the immune response. These are ABO blood group antigens, HLA antigens and minor histocompatibility antigens. Blood group compatibility is mandatory. HLA matching is beneficial, but minor antigen matching is currently not possible.

ABO blood group compatibility is a prerequisite for successful renal transplantation. Grafting across the ABO blood group barrier results in acute irreversible vascular rejection within hours or days, due to the presence of pre-existing natural blood group antibodies reactive with A and/or B antigens present on donor kidney endothelium. Reports of successful ABO incompatible grafts may be a consequence of a lack of high-titre antibodies in the recipient. One exception is the successful transplantation of blood group A2 kidneys into O recipients due to the low immunogenicity of A determinants on A2 kidneys. The combined use of pretransplant donor-specific platelet transfusions, recipient splenectomy and plasmapheresis enables the use of live related ABO incompatible donors, but such procedures are not widely practised. Organ exchange organizations aim to transplant within identical blood group types, so as to diminish the disadvantage to blood group type O recipients, who can only receive blood group type O kidneys.

2. Cell surface glycoproteins encoded for by genes of the major histocompatibility complex (MHC), termed HLA in humans, are central to the development of a specific immune response. Foreign antigens in the form of processed peptides are presented to the T-cell receptor (TCR) in association with self MHC molecules (MHC restriction). The HLA region maps to the short arm of chromosome 6 and spans 4 million base pairs of DNA with over 200 recognized genes, many with unknown functions. It has traditionally been divided into three major clusters which exhibit a remarkable degree of genetic polymorphism.

The class I genes code for the classical transplantation antigens HLA-A, B and C, which are expressed on the majority of nucleated cells. They play a central role in the binding and presentation of peptides derived from cytoplasmic proteins to CD8+ (cytotoxic) T cells. The class II genes code for the HLA-D region products HLA-DR, DQ and DP, which are constitutively expressed on antigen-presenting cells (APC) of bone marrow origin (B cells, monocytes, macrophages, dendritic cells). Following induction by cytokines their tissue range becomes more extensive. Most CD4+ helper T cells recognize peptides derived from endocytosed proteins in association with class II products. Class I and II molecules have a similar structure with an antigen-binding cleft formed by a floor of beta-pleated sheets and side walls of alpha-helices. The HLA genes are extremely polymorphic; almost all the sequence variation between HLA alleles is located in the peptide-binding groove. Different peptides derived from the same proteins bind to different HLA alleles.

In parallel with elucidation of the structure and function of the MHC, it was recognized that tumour/graft rejection was under genetic control and mapped to the MHC region and that graft rejection in humans correlated with mismatching of the gene products of the HLA region. Non-self HLA (allo) antigens induce uniquely strong primary immune responses, leading to allograft rejection.

3. The HLA gene products are co-dominantly expressed and the genes on one chromosome are inherited *en bloc* and represent an HLA haplotype. An individual inherits one maternal and one paternal haplotype. The probability of having an HLA-identical sibling is 25% and of sharing one haplotype with a sibling is 50%. Recombination events within the MHC are about 1%. The probability of finding an HLA-identical unrelated individual is very small due to enormous polymorphisms of the HLA system. The frequencies of alleles vary within a population and between different ethnic groups.

   Linkage disequilibrium refers to the phenomenon whereby certain allele associations (haplotypes) occur more often than would be predicted by chance. Such haplotypes may be frequent (A1 B8 DR3) or rare (A1 B37 DR10). Mechanisms for the generation of polymorphism remain controversial but are functionally important, occurring around the peptide-binding cleft. They are thought to be selected for on the basis that they confer functional advantages in the generation of an immune response. The presence of a large number of alleles within a population ensures the generation of an effective immune response against a wide variety of antigens.

4. Serological and molecular methods are currently employed for prospective HLA typing for renal transplants.

   The *microlymphocytotoxicity* assay utilizing serological reagents (allo-antisera and, more recently, monoclonal antibodies) has played an important role in the detection of HLA polymorphisms. This technique has been universally employed for HLA-A, B, C, DR and DQ typing. The National Institutes of Health (NIH) protocol is accepted as the standard procedure with local modifications. The assay is a three-stage complement-dependent reaction in which viable lymphocytes are incubated with HLA-specific antibody. Rabbit serum as a complement source is added; antibody bound to HLA antigens activates the complement pathway, resulting in cell death which is assessed by light microscopy. Several hundred antisera are required to obtain a complete single HLA phenotype. Obtaining useful allo-antisera requires extensive and expensive screening procedures. The operational specificity of antibodies is dependent on many factors (relating to source of complement, cell viability, antigen expression) and requires skill and experience in the interpretation of results. Due to its limitations of resolution and reproducibility, serological analysis of HLA types is rapidly being replaced with molecular typing procedures.

The application of molecular methods has resulted in a fundamental change in class II typing and is likely to result in the same for class I in the near future. *Restriction fragment length polymorphism* (RFLP) analysis of genomic DNA was shown to correlate with HLA-DR types. Limitations exist due to the failure to discriminate between certain alleles which have identical RFLP patterns. Reports show a 20% discrepancy between RFLP and serologically defined HLA-DR assignments due to difficulties associated with serological methods. Time constraints do not allow this method to be used for prospective cadaveric matching.

The *polymerase chain reaction* (PCR) in which HLA genes are selectively amplified is a technique that achieves high specificity and can be used for prospective matching. Individual alleles can be identified with the use of sequence-specific oligonucleotides (SSO) which are complementary to different motifs within the hypervariable HLA sequences. The choice of PCR-based methods that are utilized will depend on sample throughput, clinical urgency and resolution requirements.

5. The clinical usefulness of HLA-matching is dependent upon the nature of the transplant. In renal transplantation between HLA-identical siblings the benefit of matching is

generally accepted, with reported graft survival of 25 years compared to 13 years for haplotype-matched sibling grafts. A positive effect of HLA matching in cadaveric transplants is shown in most multicentre studies. Some single-centre studies show no effect of matching and may result from the low number of well-matched transplants analysed or optimization of other transplant variables.

Collaborative transplant studies reveal a beneficial effect of matching for individual loci, HLA-A, B and DR, and a stepwise decline in graft survival with an increase in the number of HLA mismatches. One-year survival of well-matched cadaveric transplants shows a difference of 10–20% graft survival when compared to highly mismatched combinations. Six-antigen-matching yields a significant improvement in 1-year graft survival rate (88%) and long-term graft survival rates (17-year half-life) in first-time recipients of HLA-A, B and DR-matched cadaver–donor grafts, when compared with first-time recipients of mismatched grafts (79%, 7.8 years respectively).

Consensus on the importance of matching for the different HLA loci has not been reached. The significant effects of matching for HLA-DR may be more pronounced in the first few months. Matching for HLA-B may have a more pronounced effect than matching for HLA-A. Eurotransplant have a hierachy of matching HLA-DR > B > A, but other centres may have a different emphasis. On an individual patient basis, clinical urgency and sensitization may override the requirements for HLA matching.

Prospective matching for other transplanted organs has not yet been fully introduced, although retrospective studies for heart transplantation show an effect of matching on graft survival and incidence of rejection episodes.

6. Hyperacute rejection is inevitable for patients with circulating cytotoxic donor-specific HLA antibodies. Development of alloantibodies may result from pregnancies, blood transfusions or transplantation. The nature of the antibody response is dependent on the method of alloantigen presentation. Alloantibodies are usually immunoglobulin G (IgG) but transient IgM can be detected following blood transfusions or transplantation.

   (a) Circulating IgG or IgM class I donor-specific cytotoxic antibodies in the current sera are a contraindication to transplantation.

(b) There is evidence to suggest that transplants with historical positive IgG class I donor-specific cross-matches should be avoided. (The relevance of such antibodies is a point of debate; some centres disregard them and claim no reduction in graft survival.)

(c) If shown to be transient, historical IgM donor-specific antibodies are not thought to be relevant.

(d) Current HLA class II donor-specific cytotoxic antibodies are sometimes, but not always, associated with hyperacute rejection and some centres avoid them.

(e) Some centres perform a cross-match using *flow cytometry*, which can detect non-complement-fixing antibodies and is more sensitive than *lymphocytotoxic cross-matching*. The value of this added sensitivity is not yet clear.

(f) A positive cross-match due to autoantibodies (usually IgM) may not result in graft failure, but they need to be carefully identified prior to transplantation.

Due to the requirement for a negative cross-match, highly sensitized patients are difficult to transplant. Identification of alloantibody specificity and measurement of antibodies present against a panel of cells (% panel reactive antibody) is predictive of how sera may react if cross-matched against random donors. Ideally, sensitized patients should be transplanted with well-matched grafts. Retransplantation with grafts carrying HLA antigens encountered on a previously failed graft should be avoided. A policy of acceptable mismatch grafts is adopted by Eurotransplant for highly sensitized patients. Recipients who receive HLA-DR-matched grafts with a negative cross-match on historical and current sera have excellent graft survival.

Further reading

Dyer P and Middleton D. (1993) *Histocompatibility Testing – A Practical Approach*. The practical approach series. D Rickwood, BD Hames. IRL Press, Oxford

Lechler R. (1994) *HLA and Disease*. Academic Press, London

Thompson AW and Catto GRD. (1993) *Immunology of Renal Transplantation*. Edward Arnold, London

Paul Brookes
Robert I. Lechler

Case 20 Medical disease in the surgical patient: recent myocardial infarction in the context of routine elective surgery

A 65-year-old man was referred with severe intermittent claudication which limited his otherwise active lifestyle. Investigations confirmed an occlusion of his left superficial femoral artery that was suitable for an above-knee femoropopliteal bypass procedure. However, direct questioning revealed that he had had a myocardial infarction 5 months previously and that he had subsequently been suffering from attacks of syncope. An ECG indicated that the patient had complete heart block and, following referral to a cardiologist, a permanent pacemaker was implanted. Subsequently the patient underwent a femoropopliteal bypass using reversed saphenous vein, 6 months following his myocardial infarction.

One year later the patient presented with an acutely ischaemic left leg following occlusion of his femoropopliteal bypass graft. An unsuccessful attempt was made to unblock the graft with percutaneous intragraft thrombolysis and the patient proceeded to revisional surgery. A below-knee polytetrafluoroethylene graft with a distal vein cuff was successful in revascularizing the limb. The patient developed acute pulmonary oedema 24 h postoperatively and, despite the absence of chest pain, a 12-lead ECG confirmed an acute myocardial infarction. The patient was transferred to the coronary care unit where he died 4 h later. Postmortem confirmed a massive myocardial infarction.

Questions

1. How long should surgery be delayed following a myocardial infarction, and why?
2. What clinical factors increase the risk of a perioperative cardiac event? How may this risk be quantified?
3. What preoperative investigations may be used to assess the severity of cardiac disease?
4. In patients considered to be at high risk of cardiac complications from their surgery, what precautions can be taken to minimize risk?

5. What specific precautions should be taken during surgery in patients who have a permanent cardiac pacemaker?
6. If it is known that a patient has had a myocardial infarction, how may this knowledge affect the choice of thrombolytic agent by a vascular surgeon or radiologist planning the treatment of acute limb ischaemia?

Answers

1. Surgery should be delayed for 6 months following myocardial infarction.

   Fewer than 0.2% of all patients undergoing surgery suffer a perioperative myocardial infarction. However, for patients who have had a previous myocardial infarction the risk of reinfarction is some 6%. Although a history of myocardial infarction is a marker of significant coronary artery disease, a number of studies have also shown that the risk of reinfarction is specifically related to the interval between the initial cardiac event and surgery. Thus, if surgery is performed 0–3 months post myocardial infarction, the risk is 30–100%. This reduces to about 15% 4–6 months post myocardial infarction and to 5% when the interval is greater than 6 months.

   Surprisingly, myocardial infarction is more likely to occur 24–48 h postoperatively than intraoperatively. Furthermore, chest pain is often absent. Patients may therefore present with hypotension, pulmonary oedema or an arrhythmia. In the elderly, unexplained confusion may be related to a reduction in cardiac output.

   The mechanism by which surgery precipitates reinfarction is unclear but rupture of coronary artery plaque, coronary artery spasm and intraluminal thrombosis may be influenced by perioperative events. These include increased blood viscosity, platelet aggregation and coronary artery spasm secondary to the humoral stress response to surgery and an increase in circulating inflammatory mediators.

   Both angina (8%) and silent myocardial ischaemia (40%) are also common during the perioperative period in patients with coronary artery disease, as are cardiac failure (5%) and arrhythmias (80%). Cardiac failure is more likely to occur within 60 min of surgery and is usually due to fluid overload on a background of impaired cardiac reserve and myocardial depression by anaesthetic agents. It may also occur 24–48 h postoperatively following the mobilization of sequestered interstitial fluid.

The incidence of clinically significant arrhythmias is approximately 5%. Myocardial ischaemia, electrolyte imbalance, increased sympathetic tone, circulating adrenergic hormones and inflammatory mediators may all promote these.

2. More than 100 studies have attempted to identify predictors of an adverse cardiac outcome following surgery but the results are conflicting. Only three undisputed factors have emerged: history of myocardial infarction, significant heart failure (with S3 gallop or raised jugular venous pressure) and surgery that involves cross-clamping of the abdominal aorta.

Coronary artery disease is almost certainly a predictor of cardiac complications but the symptoms of coronary artery disease (angina, heart block, arrhythmia) do not emerge as positive risk factors from multivariate analyses because coronary artery disease is so often silent. Similarly, whilst only 8% of patients undergoing peripheral vascular surgery have normal coronary angiograms and up to 15% suffer a perioperative myocardial infarction, peripheral vascular disease does not emerge as an independent risk factor because it is present in many elderly patients undergoing non-vascular surgery. Other factors that should increase awareness as to the possibility of cardiac complications include old age, hypertension, diabetes, smoking, hyperlipidaemia, aortic stenosis and mitral regurgitation.

Multivariate analysis has been used by Goldman *et al.* (1977) to identify, weight and score nine predictors of an adverse cardiac outcome. The scores are summed to produce a cardiac risk index that allows patients to be stratified into four levels of risk, although neither this nor other scoring systems have proved consistent.

3. Since clinical factors are unreliable indicators of cardiac risk, investigations of varying sophistication and invasiveness have been used to identify high-risk patients. Routine 12-lead ECG and chest X-ray are normal in 30% of patients with coronary artery disease and are thus of limited value. Similarly, exercise testing and precordial or transoesophageal echocardiography have a low sensitivity. Ambulatory

ECG monitoring and dipyramidol thallium imaging have shown promise, the latter having a specificity of up to 96%, although they are impractical for the majority of patients. The morbidity and cost of cardiac catheterization make its use inappropriate except in a small proportion of patients thought to be at particularly high risk because of a poor cardiac history, or in patients undergoing a major vascular procedure (e.g. thoracoabdominal aneurysm repair). Several algorithms have been suggested by which high-risk patients are identified and subjected to coronary angiography, low-risk patients proceed to surgery and intermediate-risk patients undergo further investigations. However, intensive preoperative investigation has not been proven to have a beneficial effect on outcome. Thus preoperative assessment should probably be limited to 12-lead ECG and chest X-ray with further investigations only in those patients who have symptoms that would justify them in their own right, or in patients being considered for particularly high-risk surgery.

4. Potentially correctable abnormalities, such as cardiac failure, arrhythmias, conduction abnormalities, hypertension and chronic obstructive airways disease should be identified and treatment initiated preoperatively. If coronary artery bypass grafting (CABG) or coronary angioplasty is indicated, it should be performed before other surgery except, perhaps, carotid endarterectomy. For patients who require both CABG and carotid endarterectomy, the two operations may be performed as a combined procedure.

In most cases elective surgery should be delayed to allow optimal treatment of significant medical conditions. Patients should also be encouraged to stop smoking and to reduce their weight if appropriate. In addition to its chronic effects, smoking may also increase platelet aggregation, induce coronary artery spasm and reduce the oxygen-carrying capacity of the blood secondary to elevated carboxyhaemoglobin levels. There is, however, no firm evidence that any of these measures affects outcome as controlled trials are not possible.

Perioperative fluctuations in blood pressure almost certainly contribute to peroperative cardiac morbidity, with episodes of hypotension being particularly hazardous. Attempts should be made to maintain haemodynamic equilibrium and high-risk patients should be monitored with intra-arterial blood pressure and central venous pressure measurements. The role of pulmonary artery pressure monitoring in reducing risk is unclear. Theoretically the choice of inhalation anaesthetic may be important, as agents differ in the degree of myocardial depression and hypotension that they produce, although there is no convincing evidence to support this concept. Similarly, whilst it has not been shown that there is a difference in cardiac morbidity between regional and general anaesthesia, it is generally accepted that spinal anaesthesia should be avoided in patients with a fixed cardiac output because of its vasodilatory effects. It is also essential that hypotension and hypoxia are avoided in the postoperative period as this is when the majority of cardiac events occur.

5. The use of diathermy may compromise both the sensing and pacing functions of a permanent pacemaker either by producing electromagnetic interference which inhibits the pacemaker or by conducting current down the pacing leads to produce endocardial burns. Although the response of the pacemaker to diathermy depends upon the type and its settings, the easiest way of preventing complications is to avoid the use of diathermy whenever possible. Whilst bipolar diathermy is much less likely to interfere with a pacemaker, there still remains a small risk. In circumstances where the use of diathermy is obligatory the diathermy electrodes should be placed as far from the pacemaker as possible and diathermy should be used in short bursts (1 s duration) 10 s apart. It is essential that heart rate is monitored continuously and, since diathermy often causes interference on the ECG monitor, a pulse oximeter or intra-arterial blood pressure trace should also be used. Some pacemakers can be temporarily programmed with a toroid magnet to pace continuously, making them immune to diathermy interference. In others the combination of magnet and electromagnetic interference can have disastrous effects on the programming and thus advice should be sought from the cardiology department, and pacemaker function checked both before and after surgery.

6. Thrombolysis is an established therapy for myocardial infarction. Similarly, it is used with increasing frequency as first-line therapy in a proportion of patients with acute limb ischaemia. Of the three thrombolytic agents in common use – streptokinase, anistreplase and tissue plasminogen

activator (t-PA) – only t-PA is non-antigenic. After administration of either streptokinase of anistreplase a rise in antibody titre reduces the efficacy of subsequent doses of these drugs and increases the risk of an allergic reaction. Titres remain high for up to 1 year. Thus if either agent has been used within this time, t-PA is the agent of choice for further thrombolysis.

References and further reading

Goldman L, Caldera D, Southwick F et al. (1977) Multifactorial index of cardiac risk in non cardiac surgical procedures. *New England Journal of Medicine* **297:** 845–857

Jalil S and Morris GK. (1990) Antistreptokinase titres after intravenous streptokinase. *Lancet* **335:** 184–185

Mangano DT. (1990) Peri-operative cardiac morbidity. *Anaesthesia* **72:** 153–161

Merli GJ and Weitz HH. (1992) *Medical Management of the Surgical Patient.* WB Saunders, Philadelphia

Roizen MF. (1992) Anaesthetic complications of concurrent diseases. In: Miller R (ed.) *Anaesthesia,* 4th edn. Churchill Livingstone, Edinburgh

A.J. McCleary
Michael J. Gough

Case 21 Massive rectal bleeding

A 70-year-old man presented to accident and emergency following a large passage of bright red blood from the rectum. Abdominal examination was unremarkable but the patient was hypotensive (blood pressure 90/60 mmHg) and had a tachycardia of 110 beats/min.

Questions

1. What is the likely diagnosis?
2. What is the incidence and aetiology?
3. How would you prove the diagnosis?
4. How would you manage this patient?

Answers

1. Diverticular disease is one of the more common causes of massive lower gastrointestinal bleeding.

   Most patients with diverticular haemorrhage present with only minor or occult bleeding; 50% of patients give a history of a previous episode of colonic haemorrhage.

   With the advent of improved localization techniques, angiodysplastic lesions, also known as arteriovenous malformations, have been implicated with increasing frequency as a cause of colonic bleeding. Other causes include colonic neoplasms, inflammatory bowel disease, ischaemic colitis and rare congenital lesions.

   Since as many as 30–40% of patients with lower intestinal haemorrhage never have the site of bleeding accurately determined, there is significant variation in the reported incidence of diverticular bleeding.
2. Bleeding can be expected to develop in 15% of patients with diverticulosis. Diverticular haemorrhage arises from the right colon in 70–90% of patients; this may be related to the thinner wall of the right colon. Approximately 70% of patients with diverticular haemorrhage cease bleeding spontaneously; the risk of rebleeding is only 30% but increases to 50% in patients who have suffered a second episode of haemorrhage.

Diverticular haemorrhage is thought to follow injury and subsequent rupture of blood vessels lying adjacent to a diverticulum. Diverticula develop at potential weak points in the colonic wall where the nutrient blood vessels penetrate the circular muscle layer en route to the mucosa. As a diverticulum begins to herniate, it tends to carry one of the penetrating vessels with it. Eventually the vessel becomes draped over the dome of the diverticulum, separated from the colonic lumen only by the thin mucosal layer. This anatomical relationship predisposes to injury with subsequent rupture. Characteristic pathological changes in the vasa recta of bleeding diverticula have been observed, namely eccentric thickening of the intima and thinning of the underlying media. In all cases, rupture occurs eccentrically into the lumen of the diverticulum.

3. One-third of patients with diverticular haemorrhage present with massive exsanguinating haemorrhage. The first step is immediate resuscitation. The passage of a nasogastric tube helps to exclude an upper gastrointestinal source of bleeding. Resuscitation should precede any further diagnostic manoeuvres.

All patients should undergo proctoscopy as soon as possible to exclude the rectum as the bleeding source. Identification of bleeding from haemorrhoids or other rectal lesions is extremely important as a differential diagnosis.

In total, 70–80% of patients stop bleeding spontaneously and should undergo elective evaluation.

Continued massive bleeding in a haemodynamically unstable patient is an indication for emergency surgical intervention with on-table panendoscopy of the gastrointestinal tract. In actively bleeding patients who maintain relative haemodynamic stability, attempts at localization of the bleeding site should be made by selective mesenteric arteriography, radioactive scanning or colonoscopy. Selective mesenteric angiography successfully identifies the site of haemorrhage in 40–60% of patients.

In order for arteriography to be successful, bleeding must be ongoing at a minimal rate of 0.5 ml/min; limiting arteriography to such patients produces a diagnostic yield of 70–100%. Another alternative, even in the actively bleeding patient, is to perform diagnostic colonoscopy, although visualization may be difficult.

Radioisotope scans are of two basic types: ^{99m}Tc-labelled sulphur colloid or red blood cells. ^{99m}Tc sulphur colloid, once injected intravenously, is cleared from the circulation by the liver, spleen and bone marrow within several minutes. Any labelled colloid that extravasates into the intestinal lumen is not cleared and remains, it is hoped, near the site of bleeding. Any abnormal radioactive pooling can be detected on scanning. The study is completed within a short time, and bleeding rates as low as 0.1 ml/min can be detected reliably. Labelled erythrocytes, however, have a relatively long half-life within the circulation. Scanning can be repeated at 24 or 36 h after injection – a useful tool in the detection of chronic or intermittent bleeding.

Although accurate in the detection of active bleeding, radioisotope scans have had variable success in accurately localizing the site of haemorrhage. In one series of 59 patients, the site of bleeding was suggested in 36 (61%) but in only 25 patients (42%) did the activity on scintigraphy correlate with an actual pathological lesion demonstrated by other means (endoscopy, angiography or surgical therapy). Others have reported localization accuracy rates of 24–81%.

One reason for the relatively poor localization rates is that blood within the intestinal lumen does not remain stationary. For example, blood originally extravasated into the caecum may pass rapidly into the distal colon after only a few peristaltic waves. Similarly, with an incompetent ileocaecal valve, blood may reflux proximally into the small intestine. In either case, subsequent scanning may not determine accurate localization. Normal anatomical relationships may also be responsible for diagnostic errors. Bleeding lesions in the upper gastrointestinal tract may be superimposed on adjacent colon, thereby suggesting, incorrectly, a diagnosis of colonic haemorrhage. Similarly, lesions in the transverse colon, although an unusual site of haemorrhage, may be interpreted as an upper gastrointestinal bleeding source. Bleeding from a redundant loop of sigmoid colon, which drapes towards the patient's right lower quadrant, may be falsely identified as bleeding from the right colon. For all these reasons, segmental colon resection based solely upon the results of a positive bleeding scan should be undertaken with caution.

Despite the wide variations noted, such scans are frequently obtained as the initial diagnostic study in patients with intestinal haemorrhage. Currently, several centres utilize nuclear scanning as a screening test to determine the need for subsequent arteriography. Patients with positive red cell scans proceed to selective arteriography, whereas those with no evidence of active bleeding are observed for signs of further haemorrhage. Red cell scans are extremely sensitive in detecting active bleeding, with false-negative and false-positive rates of less than 10%. By reserving arteriography for the patient with a positive scan, the diagnostic accuracy of this study can be substantially improved, often to greater than 90%.

In patients who have ceased bleeding, diagnostic studies can be performed on a more elective basis. The colon should be adequately prepared and colonoscopy performed with excellent mucosal visualization. Elective colonoscopy should have a diagnostic sensitivity of 90% in detecting non-bleeding lesions of the colon. The double-contrast barium enema is still a useful test but may have a sensitivity of only 70% in this situation. This test should rarely, if ever, be obtained in the early diagnostic period as, when barium contrast has been introduced into the colon, it obscures any subsequent attempts to visualize the colonic lumen by arteriography or colonoscopy.

4. Initial resuscitative measures, as for any patient with gastro-intestinal haemorrhage and hypovolaemia, should be instituted promptly. With adequate fluid resuscitation, blood transfusion and correction of coagulation abnormalities, 70–80% of patients cease bleeding spontaneously. However, approximately 15% of all patients presenting with massive diverticular haemorrhage require emergency surgical intervention before further diagnostic information can be obtained. The mortality in this group is high, often approaching 30–50%.

    Emergency surgical intervention is recommended in any patient who continues to bleed despite all resuscitative and therapeutic manoeuvres. Indications for emergent operation include persistent haemodynamic instability and recurrent haemorrhage. Emergency surgical therapy can be either directed or non-directed, depending on the success or failure of preoperative localization. If a bleeding site has been identified by colonoscopy, arteriography or nuclear scanning, a segmental resection can be performed with the expectation that bleeding is controlled in over 90% of patients. If the source of bleeding has not been identified, on-table colonic lavage with panendoscopy of the entire gastrointestinal tract is recommended. Emergency subtotal colectomy without preoperative localization of the bleeding site has an operative mortality of 30–50% with angiographic localization and a more limited resection; an operative mortality of 20–30% can be expected with emergency intervention. This can be reduced to less than 10% when surgical therapy is performed on an elective basis. Segmental resection or hemicolectomy should not be performed when the site of colonic haemorrhage has not been identified. Such procedures are associated with an extremely high rate of rebleeding (35–50%) and an increased operative mortality (30%), as compared with the rates of rebleeding (10%) and mortality (10%) after subtotal colectomy.

Ravinder Singh Nagra
W. Kmiot

Case 22 Postoperative jaundice

A slim 24-year-old woman undergoes a laparoscopic cholecystectomy following several attacks of colicky pain associated with multiple small gallstones. Her preoperative liver function tests were normal and no intraoperative cholangiogram was performed. The procedure appeared to be straightforward, except that the gallbladder was torn at Hartmann's pouch by the grasping forceps with spillage of bile and small stones, most of which were retrieved. The following morning the patient was complaining of upper abdominal and right shoulder-tip pain and she vomited after eating a light breakfast. On examination there was only mild upper abdominal tenderness and low-grade fever (37.8°). She had a white blood cell count of 14 000/mm^3. She was kept in hospital and her symptoms remained unchanged. However, by the second postoperative day she was noted to have scleral icterus. This had deepened by day 3 and her liver function tests were as given in Table 22.1.

Table 22.1

		Normal range
Bilirubin	70 μmol/l	3–17 μmol/l
Alkaline phosphatase	400 iu/l	3–300 iu/l
Aspartate aminotransferase	45 iu/l	5–35 iu/l
Alanine aminotransferase	52 iu/l	5–35 iu/l
Glutamyl transpeptidase	150 iu/l	11–51 iu/l

Questions

1. What is the differential diagnosis in this case?
2. Apart from repeating the liver function tests, list in order the investigations you would do and what information you would be looking for.
3. What would be the preferred management of a small obstructing common bile duct stone in this case?
4. List the types of injury to the biliary tree that may occur during laparoscopic cholecystectomy. What is the estimated incidence of such injuries?

5. What would be the management of choice in each of the following situations?
   (a) An intraperitoneal bile collection without apparent continuing leakage.
   (b) Cystic duct stump leakage due to a slipped clip.
   (c) Complete occlusion of the common hepatic duct by a clip.
   (d) Late mid-duct stricture with cholangitis at 6 months following resolution of the early problems.
6. How can we minimize the risk of biliary injuries at laparoscopic cholecystectomy?

Answers

1. The differential diagnosis is:
   (a) Bile duct injuries: these are the most serious biliary complication of laparoscopic cholecystectomy. The incidence of these injuries is probably at least twice that following the open procedure. It is estimated that 0.6–0.7% of patients having laparoscopic cholecystectomy will have significant bile duct injury.
   (b) Retained common bile duct stones: this will occur in about 0.3–0.7% of patients having laparoscopic cholecystectomy, a figure very similar to that following the open procedure. It is feared, however, that bile duct stones are missed more frequently at laparoscopic cholecystectomy, which may lead to a higher incidence of retained stones in the future.
   (c) Bile leakage: this may result in the formation of localized biloma, bile peritonitis or bile fistula. The incidence is similar following both laparoscopic and open cholecystectomy.
2. Ultrasonography and computed tomography (CT) can be used to visualize intra- and extrahepatic bile duct dilatation and fluid collection. Cholangiography is the investigation of choice if either of the above modalities shows dilatation of the biliary tree. It is performed either by the endoscopic route (endoscopic retrograde cholangiopancreatography, ERCP), or the percutaneous route (percutaneous transhepatic cholangiography, PTC).
   Cholangiography is useful in demonstrating retained

calculi, bile leakage, strictures and distal obstruction. It also has the advantage of being a therapeutic tool; the endoscopist can remove retained stones or place transhepatic stents for external decompression in obstructive jaundice.

Radionuclide scanning (HIDA) is very accurate in detecting bile leakage and bile duct obstruction but poor definition of the anatomy of the injury is a disadvantage.

3. The preferred procedure for removing a small stone which is obstructing the common bile duct is endoscopic sphincterotomy. This is very effective and success rates over 95% have been reported in highly selected patients. The procedure entails the introduction of a duodenoscope which facilitates the insertion of a guidewire and a catheter into the common bile duct. A sphincterotomy is performed and the stone is either actively removed by passing a balloon-tipped catheter or a basket and extracting it, or it is left to pass spontaneously.

Complications occur in about 5–10% of patients. These include bleeding, pancreatitis, cholangitis and retroperitoneal perforation, for which urgent surgery is needed in 1–2% of cases. The overall mortality of endoscopic sphincterotomy, which is related to the age and the general condition of the patient, is estimated at 1–1.5%.

4. The most common biliary complication of laparoscopic cholecystectomy is a leak from the cystic duct due either to poor application of the clip, or the use of electrocautery near metal clips.

Injuries to the biliary tree at laparoscopic cholecystectomy may involve any part of the tree and may be due to laceration, excision or occlusion of the duct. In the most serious injury the common bile duct is mistaken for the cystic duct and excised with the gallbladder. If the surgeon continues upward dissection on the medial aspect of the common bile duct and the hepatic duct, the right hepatic artery may also be injured. Complete or partial obstruction of the common bile duct may occur as a result of application of a clip to the duct.

Strictures (sometimes presenting weeks to months after operation) may occur as a result of different factors, including thermal injury, infection or devascularization. Strictures are classified according to the Bismuth scale into four grades. Grade I strictures are more than 2 cm from the confluence of the right and left hepatic duct; grade II are less than 2 cm from the confluence but a remnant of a common hepatic duct exists, in grade III there is no remnant of the common hepatic duct and in grade IV there is loss of continuity between the right and left hepatic ducts.

The incidence of bile duct injuries following laparoscopic cholecystectomy has been estimated (in a large survey of surgeons in the USA) at about 0.6%. A well-controlled prospective study from the UK puts the incidence at 0.7%, which is twice as high as bile duct injuries following the open procedure.

5. (a) An intraperitoneal bile collection without continuing leakage is treated by percutaneous drainage employing either ultrasound or CT scanning. The aspirate is cultured and tested for antibiotic sensitivity. Drainage is always performed under antibiotic cover and the catheter is flushed three to four times a day with normal saline to prevent occlusion with bile.

   (b) The treatment of cystic duct stump leakage due to slipped clip is endoscopic stenting of the bile duct. The stent is inserted under antibiotic cover to a level higher than the orifice of the cystic duct into the common bile duct, thus occluding the cystic duct. The stent may be removed after several weeks.

   (c) Complete occlusion of the common bile duct by a clip requires reoperation. While excision of the affected area and an end-to-end anastomosis are occasionally successful, a Roux-en-Y hepaticojejunostomy is the treatment of choice, especially in the presence of gross soiling, or if an anastomosis cannot be performed without tension.

   (d) Late mid-duct stricture complicated by cholangitis: cholangitis is treated with antibiotics. The site, nature and extent of the stricture are determined by cholangiography. Surgical management with a Roux-en-Y hepaticojejunostomy is the treatment of choice in most cases. Endoscopic balloon dilatation is often useful but may prove ineffective in the long term because of recurrent stricture formation.

6. In order to minimize the incidence of untoward accidents it is important for surgeons intending to practise laparoscopic surgery to acquire thorough training.

   Adequate insufflation, exposure of the biliary tree by careful dissection of Calot's triangle and traction on Hartmann's pouch in the direction of the right iliac fossa (to bring the cystic duct perpendicular to the common hepatic duct) are fundamentals of safe laparoscopic cholecystectomy. The use of a 30° laparoscope will help surgeons to obtain the more familiar vertical view of the anatomy.

The use of diathermy should be restricted to areas away from the bile duct and the hilum of the liver. Diathermy should never be used near a metal clip. The use of an intra-operative cholangiogram remains a controversial issue; however, when used with fluoroscopy it is useful in showing the biliary anatomy and demonstrating leaks.

Difficulties may arise as a result of technical failure, poor vision, unfamiliarity with the frequently anomalous anatomy, extensive inflammation and scarring, and in the obese patient. In such cases in order to minimize the risk of bile duct injury the surgeon should use his or her judgement and have a low threshold to abandon the procedure and convert to the open one.

Further reading

Fletcher DR. (1993) Biliary injury at laparoscopic cholecystectomy: recognition and prevention. *Australia and New Zealand Journal of Surgery* **63:** 673–677

Fullarton GM and Bell G. (1994) Prospective audit of the introduction of laparoscopic cholecystectomy in the west of Scotland. *Gut* **35**(8): 1121–1126

Raute M, Podlech P, Jaschke W *et al.* (1993) Management of bile duct injuries and strictures following cholecystectomy. *World Journal of Surgery* **17:** 553–562

Reyad Al-Ghnaniem
Irving S. Benjamin

Case 23 Aggressive peptic ulceration

A 40-year-old man who had undergone a vagotomy for duodenal ulcer suffered a recurrent painful ulcer not responsive to treatment. At an operation for haemorrhage an inflammatory peripyloric ulcer mass was avoided by performing an antrectomy and Billroth II (Polya) partial gastrectomy. Soon afterwards he developed a stomal ulcer, confirmed on endoscopy, and complained of diarrhoea.

Questions

1. What two main diagnoses should be considered?
2. What investigations should be performed?
3. What are the complications of stomal ulcer?
4. What alternative treatments would have been considered at the time of his original bleeding duodenal ulcer?
5. What are the principles of management of the Zollinger–Ellison syndrome (ZES)?

Answers

1. ZES and retained antrum. The latter should never be forgotten as a possibility when a gastrectomy has been performed in a patient with an inflammatory mass, when the antrectomy may be incomplete. The retained antrum is excluded from the acid stream, and produces excess gastrin as a result.

   In ZES gastrin is secreted from a gastrinoma, situated most commonly in the pancreas, but sometimes in the duodenum or stomach. Rarely such tumours are in lymph nodes or even the ovary or parathyroid. About one-third of patients will have evidence of multiple endocrine neoplasia, usually in the form of hyperparathyroidism.
2. Plasma gastrin should be assayed. It would be raised in both conditions. The highest gastrins are found in achlorhydria (50–100 × normal) rather than in ZES. The levels in retained antrum are above normal, but depend on the amount of

central tissue remaining. Ultrasound and computed tomographic (CT) scanning are important tools for localizing a gastrinoma, being successful in about 80% of cases.

Gastric acid secretion may be measured. In both cases basal secretion will be raised. In ZES secretion may be very high, but the basal/stimulated secretion ratio is particularly high.

3. Stomal ulcers are high-risk ulcers. They commonly bleed, and because of the anatomical rearrangements associated with partial gastrectomy tend to penetrate into the transverse colon, producing a gastrocolic fistula. Such fistulas present with severe diarrhoea, which results from small-bowel colonization (via the fistula) with colonic flora. This was once treated by an initial diverting colostomy, but today appropriate antibiotic therapy may be followed by definitive treatment.

A fistula is treated by resection; in the absence of fistulation stomal ulcers will respond to treatment with a proton-pump inhibitor, but because recurrence is frequent and dangerous such treatment must be considered permanent, or alternatively as preparation for surgery. In the absence of ZES, surgical treatment can consist of higher gastric resection or of vagotomy. Vagotomy for such ulcers can be performed thoracoscopically, but it must be remembered that thoracic vagotomy has been found to be followed by a higher recurrent ulcer rate than abdominal vagotomy. Such operations must therefore be performed with meticulous care.

4. During an acute bleed diagnosis is confirmed at endoscopy, and endoscopic therapy should always be considered before surgery. There are three endoscopic modalities to choose from – laser coagulation, heat probe or injection therapy.

Controlled trials have indicated that the laser offers no advantage over the much cheaper heat probe. Injection therapy is the simplest, and in some series controls bleeding initially in over 80% of cases. The re-bleeding incidence is lowered by sclerotherapy, as is the need for subsequent laparotomy. Overall mortality can be lowered by such an approach. The agent used for injection may be 1:10 000 adrenaline or alcohol.

5. ZES is diagnosed when a patient with aggressive peptic ulceration is shown to have a raised fasting plasma gastrin

on radioimmunoassay, and other rare causes have been excluded, particularly retained antrum in a postoperative patient, and antral G-cell hyperplasia. Gastric hypersecretion, as indicated earlier, should be demonstrable. Tumour localization with CT and ultrasound may be supplemented by visceral angiography. Metastases in the liver are similarly confirmed or excluded.

Management is directed at the effects of hypergastrinaemia, and of the tumour. In most centres a single tumour would indicate need for a laparotomy; successful surgical removal may then cure the disease. In young patients particularly this chance should not be overlooked.

Multiple tumours, or the presence of metastases, shift the management emphasis to the target organ – the hypersecreting stomach. Total gastrectomy was once performed as almost a standard measure; since the advent of proton-pump inhibitors of gastric acid secretion (omeprazole, lansoprazole) this is no longer necessary. Satisfactory control can be achieved in almost all patients.

Metastatic disease, usually hepatic, may dominate the picture, and is managed by cytotoxic therapy (streptozotocin), tumour embolization or surgical resections to reduce tumour bulk.

Further reading

Maton PN. (1993) Review article: the management of Zollinger–Ellison syndrome. *Alimentary and Pharmacological Therapy* **7:** 467–475

Report of a joint working group of the British Society of Gastroenterology, the Research Unit of the Royal College of Physicians of London and the Audit Unit of the Royal College of Surgeons of England (1992) Guideline for good practice in an audit of the management of upper gastrointestinal haemorrhage. *Journal of the Royal College of Physicians of London* **26:** 281–289

Steger A. (1993) Acute upper gastrointestinal bleeding. In: Bouchier IAD, Allan RN, Hodgson HJF and Keighley MRB (eds) *Gastroenterology: Clinical Science and Practice.* WB Saunders, London

Tavenor J, Smith S and Sullivan S. (1993) Gastrocolic fistula. A review of 15 cases and an update of the literature. *Journal of Clinical Gastroenterology* **16:** 189–191

John Spencer

Case 24   Acute abdomen

A 66-year-old man with rheumatoid arthritis was sent to accident and emergency by his general practitioner with a history of sudden severe upper abdominal pain, which started centrally in the epigastrium and spread across the upper abdomen. On examination he was in obvious pain, was normotensive but tachycardic and had board-like rigidity of the abdomen. A chest radiograph revealed free gas under the right hemidiaphragm. There was no other relevant previous history.

Questions

1. What is the likely diagnosis, and are there important differentials?
2. What predisposing factors should be considered?
3. What is the mortality of this condition, and who is most at risk?
4. What are the pros and cons of operative or conservative therapy?
5. If operation is preferred, what methods are available, and what ancillary procedures should be considered, and when?

Answers

1. Perforated peptic ulcer, which may be gastric or duodenal. If duodenal, the ulcer is almost always anterior. The presence of gas under the diaphragm indicates a perforated viscus, but this could be a diverticulum (usually colonic) or even a perforated appendix. In older patients stercoral perforation is not uncommon. In the absence of free gas, perforation may be mimicked by acute ulceration, by acute gallbladder disease or pancreatitis, by basal pneumonia, by myocardial infarction, by aortic dissection or leaking aneurysm. It must never be forgotten that a perforated gastric ulcer may be a carcinoma.

2. A very likely important predisposing factor in this patient is the use of non-steroidal anti-inflammatory drugs (NSAIDs). These are a very common cause of peptic ulcer complications; preparations containing protective prostaglandins reduce the incidence of complications but do not eliminate them. Steroids may both predispose to peptic ulceration and perforation, and at the same time reduce signs and symptoms, making diagnosis much more difficult.

An important question to ask in every case of complicated peptic ulcer is whether there is anything to suggest the Zollinger–Ellison syndrome (ZES), in which peptic ulcer is secondary to a gastrinoma, usually in the pancreas. Most often this is indicated by a history of aggressive, non-responsive and often repeatedly complicated peptic ulcer – all absent in this case. Less florid clues might include diarrhoea (a feature of ZES). Hypercalcaemia may indicate the presence of a parathyroid adenoma, which may or may not be part of a multiple endocrine neoplasia (MEN) syndrome in a patient with duodenal ulcer.

Although NSAID-induced ulcer is an entity in itself, the underlying cause of the majority of peptic ulcers is of course infection with *Helicobacter pylori*.

3. The overall mortality of perforated peptic ulcer is about 10%. It is much higher (c. 16%) for acute ulcers and lower (2–4%) for chronic ulcers. In perforations occurring in a medical ward it has been reported to be as high as 89%; in that series most patients were elderly men with no previous ulcer history. The most significant factor is associated disease; perforation is often a terminal event in the very ill patient. A long interval between perforation and treatment carries a high mortality. As with other acute illnesses, age is of great importance, the mortality being very low in the young and middle-aged, and much higher in the elderly.

4. In all patients resuscitative measures must be the first priority; fluid and electrolyte balance must be restored before contemplating operation.

Although most patients undergo surgery, the only controlled clinical trial comparing non-operative with operative treatment revealed no difference in overall mortality. Conservative management is therefore possible, but needs to be pursued very carefully. There are four major advantages of operation:

(a) Complete peritoneal lavage is possible.

(b) The perforation may be closed.

(c) In the case of gastric ulcer a biopsy-excision will exclude a carcinoma.

(d) A definitive procedure such as a vagotomy may be added.

The disadvantages of surgery are those of any operation in the sick, and particularly the elderly, with consequent morbidity and mortality.

Conservative therapy is particularly appropriate if clinical and radiological evidence suggests localization of the perforation, or in those too sick to be anaesthetized.

5. At laparotomy ulcers are usually closed by sutures incorporating a 'plug' of omentum. If simultaneous endoscopy is performed, a biopsy forceps may be used to draw a piece of omentum into the perforation; this produces a very effective seal with no further procedure necessary. Either of these procedures can now be performed laparoscopically, and this promises to reduce mortality.

Peritoneal lavage is an important part of the operation, whether open or endoscopic. In the case of a gastric ulcer a biopsy (often excisional) should be performed to exclude a carcinoma.

If the patient's general condition permits, and the surgeon has the necessary experience, a definitive operation may be added, such as a proximal gastric vagotomy (PGV). This reduces the ulcer rate from over 60% with simple closure to less than 5% at 3 years.

In those with little or no symptoms up to the time of perforation, operations more radical than PGV should not be employed, as any side-effects will be poorly tolerated by previously well patients. In the commoner situation of perforation in a patient with a history of severe ulcer symptoms beforehand, a definitive procedure such as a vagotomy and gastroenterostomy can be considered. Controlled evidence supports the addition of such a procedure, but such trials preceded the *Helicobacter* age of ulcer management. It is now much more reasonable to withhold definitive procedures and proceed with medical treatment subsequently, including appropriate antibiotic therapy to eliminate *Helicobacter pylori*.

In the case described, the ingested NSAIDs are more likely to have been involved in the ulcer aetiology. It is known that in such cases *Helicobacter* organisms are often not present. This raises the difficult question, still unresolved, of whether such ulcers should be treated differently, and a more aggressive surgical approach adopted in the acute situation (whether perforation or haemorrhage), particularly as in these cases NSAID therapy may need to be continued.

Further reading

Koness RJ, Cutitar M and Burchard KW. Perforated peptic ulcer. Determinants of morbidity and mortality. *Annals of Surgery* **56:** 280–284

Svanes C, Salvesen H, Stangeland L, Svanes K and Soreide O. (1993) Perforated peptic ulcer over 56 years. Time trends in patients and disease characteristics. *Gut* **34:** 1666–1671

John Spencer

Case 25 Benign breast disease/ breast abscess

A 35-year-old woman noticed a painful left breast one morning when carrying her only daughter to school. That evening, whilst undressing, she found a creamy-coloured discharge from the nipple on her underwear. She consulted her general practitioner the following day and was prescribed a course of amoxycillin 500 mg t.d.s. Three days later and obviously concerned about the possibility of cancer, she discovered a lump under her nipple and attended the casualty department requesting a surgical opinion. On examination she had an axillary temperature of 37.5°C, there was marked periareolar inflammation of the left breast and a very tender 4 cm diameter spherical mass underlying the medial aspect of the areolar.

Questions

1. What is the likely diagnosis and natural disease progression?
2. Describe the management options for this condition.
3. What is the chronic complication that often occurs and how should it be managed?
4. Briefly outline the possible causes of a nipple discharge.

Answers

1. The likely diagnosis is periductal mastitis progressing to a non-lactating breast abscess. Periductal mastitis affects young women of age 30–40 years. It is a clinical syndrome characterized by non-cyclical mastalgia, nipple discharge, nipple retraction, periareolar inflammation, non-lactating breast abscess and mamillary fistula. Patients may be affected by variable degrees of this disease process. The aetiology of periductal mastitis is not known, although it is clear that bacteriological infection often supervenes and promotes the disease. The main ducts are not dilated but surrounded by an intense inflammatory cellular response. This differentiates the condition from duct ectasia, a primary

dilatation of the major ducts of the breast, which occurs in an older age group of women. Duct ectasia is thought to be a consequence of normal involution and there is little periductal inflammation; however, bacterial infection can also ensue and produce similar clinical consequences.

Nipple retraction at the site of the diseased duct occurs early in periductal mastitis and is present in up to 75% of patients who present with periareolar inflammation. Early in the disease the retraction is slight and may not be noticed; marked retraction or nipple inversion occurs with recurrent infective episodes. Nipple discharge is present in 15–20% of patients with periductal mastitis.

Breast abscess in non-lactating breasts is now more common in the developed world than those occurring during the puerperium and the majority of the periareolar type are sequelae of periductal mastitis. The causative organisms are predominantly Gram-positive cocci, i.e. *Staphylococcus aureus* and *S. epidermidis*, but anaerobic flora such as *Bacteroides* are often isolated, particularly in association with recurrent abscess, mamillary fistulas and abscesses associated with inflammatory carcinomas. Cigarette smoking has been shown to be important in the development of non-lactating breast abscess and may predispose to anaerobic breast infection and the progression to mamillary fistula.

2. All management plans should begin with a clinical history and physical examination, not only to facilitate a diagnosis but also to determine the likelihood of any underlying pathology that needs further investigation. Clinical assessment is often limited by extreme breast tenderness. The breast may be swollen and indurated and in such cases it may not be possible to confirm or exclude the presence of an abscess by clinical examination alone.

Breast ultrasound examination is very easy to perform and readily available. It has been found to be very accurate in demonstrating the presence of an abscess collection in the acutely inflamed breast. Mammography in such cases is often not very helpful for several reasons. Adequate compression of the breast may not be possible due to extreme tenderness. As this condition often affects young women, the breast parenchyma may be very dense on mammography and may conceal an underlying abscess. The mammographic features of an abscess are not specific and can be identical to those of a carcinoma. As a general rule all patients over the age of 35 years presenting with a breast complaint should have single oblique mammography; this should be performed in cases of periductal mastitis once the acute inflammation has resolved.

Breast pain associated with periductal mastitis often resolves without any specific treatment. Periareolar inflammation is often seen in association with a tender mass and antibiotic therapy alone has been shown to be effective in resolving this stage of the disease. Antibiotics should be chosen to cover both aerobic and anaerobic organisms and recently a combination of amoxycillin and clavulanic acid (Augmentin) or a cephalosporin (e.g. cephradrine) and metronidazole have been successfully used.

The majority of patients with breast abscesses can be treated as outpatients. If the overlying skin is only erythematous and not thinned or necrotic, the patient can be managed with repeated percutaneous aspiration using a 19 G (white) needle and syringe. This should be performed under antibiotic cover. If the overlying skin is thinned, a topical local anaesthetic cream is used to anaesthetize the area; incision and drainage can then be performed. Packing of the wound following this method of abscess drainage is not usually necessary. In those patients with very large abscesses or not responding to either of the above outpatient management options, admission to hospital and a general anaesthetic are required. Formal digital exploration of the abscess cavity is performed to break down any walled-off loculi and packing of the resultant wound is usually needed. Pus should be sent for bacteriological and cytological examination, although the accuracy of the cytological aspiration is impaired by the presence of concomitant infection. A biopsy of the cavity should be taken if there is a suspicion of an underlying neoplasm.

3. A mamillary duct fistula is the commonest chronic complication of the periductal mastitis disease process. It is a communication between the skin, usually in the periareolar region, and a breast duct. Almost all arise as a complication of periductal mastitis either from spontaneous discharge of an inflammatory mass or from surgical intervention. Recent studies have shown that a mamillary sinus or fistula can be demonstrated in virtually every periareolar abscess. After incision and drainage of a non-lactating breast abscess, up

to one-third of patients will develop a clinically significant chronic mamillary fistula. It is thought that the method of treating the abscess is unlikely to have any effect on the development of such a fistula. Retraction of the nipple at the site of the involved duct is present in almost all patients.

The preferred method of surgical treatment is to excise the fistula completely with its associated duct through a circumareolar incision. The wound can be closed primarily under the appropriate antibiotic cover. A portion of the nipple skin is also excised to ensure complete removal of the diseased duct and eversion of the nipple seems to reduce the incidence of recurrence. Previously laying open the fistula tract with healing by secondary intention has been the most effective method of treatment but this produces an unsightly scar across the areolar and nipple.

4. Nipple discharge arising from single or multiple ducts is very common and rarely associated with an underlying carcinoma. Single duct discharge is likely to be more serious than multiple duct discharge. Many clinicians value the division of nipple discharge into galactorrhoea, bloody and non-bloody discharge. However, the presence of blood and/or breast milk are only two of the many factors used to aid diagnosis. Investigations commence with cytological examination of the discharge and may progress to include mammography, fine-needle aspiration biopsy and, more recently, duct endoscopy and endoscopic biopsy. The causes of nipple discharge in order of decreasing frequency are:

(a) Physiological – this is by far the most common and is usually clear or yellow; it is never blood-stained. The diagnosis is one of exclusion from other pathological causes.

(b) Ductal papilloma – this is frequently blood-stained and arises from a single duct.

(c) Periductal mastitis and duct ectasia – this usually produces a cheesy-type discharge which may be blood-stained. It may arise from more than one duct.

(d) Epithelial hyperplasia and fibrocystic disease – this typically produces a discharge that may be blood-stained from several ducts.

(e) Breast cancer – ductal carcinoma may produce any type of discharge. It is usually blood-stained, arising from a single duct and often associated with an underlying palpable mass.

(f) Galactorrhoea – a milky discharge from the nipple is
normal during pregnancy and may continue following
the cessation of breastfeeding. Outside these times
galactorrhoea may be caused by drugs (oral contra-
ceptives, tricyclic antidepressants and metoclopramide),
hyperthyroidism or hypothyroidism. Under these circumstances serum prolactin levels are normal; if the
level is elevated, a prolactin-secreting pituitary tumour
should be sought.

Further reading

Smallwood JA and Taylor I. (eds) (1990) *Benign Breast Disease*. Arnold, London

Paul Anthony Harris
Dudley Sinnett

Case 26 Testicular torsion

An 18-year-old man presented to casualty with a 3-h history of acute pain in the right hemiscrotum. There were no associated symptoms. In particular there was no history of frequency, dysuria or urethral discharge. The patient gave a history of similar shorter episodes of right-sided scrotal pain of sudden onset, short duration and rapid resolution in the preceding 12 months. On examination the patient was afebrile with a soft abdomen. Examination of the scrotum revealed that the right testicle was lying higher in the scrotum than its companion and the spermatic cord was noted to feel thicker than the left spermatic cord. The right testicle and spermatic cord were extremely tender.

Questions

1. What is the diagnosis and differential diagnosis?
2. What are the investigations and what initial management would you undertake?
3. What are the principles of surgical therapy?
4. What is the underlying abnormality leading to torsion?
5. What is the expected outcome from treatment?

Answers

1. Acute scrotal pain in a young man or male adolescent is acute torsion of the spermatic cord until proven otherwise. The rapid onset of severe unilateral scrotal pain, which often wakes the patient from sleep, is characteristic of testicular torsion. In approximately half of these patients there is an antecedent history of similar episodes of scrotal pain of shorter duration with rapid resolution which is due to intermittent torsion and detorsion of the affected testicle. Not surprisingly, patients usually recall this antecedent history after the torsion has been successfully treated. The classical physical findings are a normal temperature and a tender hemiscrotum with the affected testis lying high in the scrotum and a thickened spermatic cord. As the torsion

occurs and the spermatic cord twists up to 720°, the testis is drawn upwards and the cord becomes shorter and bulkier. A useful ancillary sign is absence of dartos muscle contraction on the affected side of the scrotum when the inner aspect of the ipsilateral thigh is stroked.

The differential diagnosis includes torsion of a testicular appendage, acute epididymo-orchitis, testicular trauma and strangulated hernia. The appendix testis (hydatid of Morgagni), which is a remnant of the Müllerian duct, is the testicular appendage which torts most commonly. The patient is usually an adolescent male and in the early stages a small tender mass may be palpated at the superior pole of an otherwise normal testis.

A characteristic blue dot may be seen through the scrotal skin at the top of the testis. Acute epididiymo-orchitis is characterized by the presence of a temperature and a history of frequency, dysuria and occasionally urethral discharge. The affected testis is hot, tender and swollen. The pain of acute epididymo-orchitis is lessened by elevating the scrotum, which relieves the traction on the spermatic cord. Testicular trauma is characterized by a clear history of recent significant scrotal trauma and a bruised scrotum with a tender testis, which is often difficult to palpate because of haematoma or due to testicular disruption in severe cases. A strangulated hernia will be associated with a tender mass above an otherwise normal testis and a preceding history of an inguinoscrotal swelling.

2. The diagnosis of testicular torsion is made on the basis of presenting symptoms and physical findings and is usually clear-cut. In addition to abdominal and scrotal examination the temperature should be measured and urine microscopy performed in casualty where possible. A normal temperature and clear urine are consistent with testicular torsion whilst a pyrexia, pyuria and bacteriuria suggest acute epididymo-orchitis. If the diagnosis remains unclear a colour Doppler ultrasound or nuclear perfusion scan will show decreased or absent blood flow in testicular torsion and enhanced blood flow in acute epididymo-orchitis.

However, these investigations will delay correction of torsion. The duration of torsion is the most crucial factor in determining outcome as the testis has a very poor tolerance for ischaemia. After 4 h of ischaemia spermatogenesis is significantly impaired. For this reason the diagnosis of testicular torsion is best confirmed by *immediate* scrotal exploration.

As there is inevitably some delay in transfer to theatre, induction of anaesthesia and preparation of the patient, it is prudent to relieve the torsion in casualty by manual detorsion of the testis. If the patient finds this too uncomfortable, manual detorsion may be undertaken after induction of anaesthesia. This can be achieved by twisting the affected testicle away from the midline. Successful manual detorsion is accompanied by a significant reduction in pain but immediate exploration should proceed as the torsion may not be completely untwisted and recurrence of the torsion may occur rapidly.

3. The patient is placed lying supine on the table and the scrotum is shaved prior to preparation with antiseptic. The scrotum, penis and lower abdomen are included in the preparation. A midline incision through the scrotal raphe is made as this allows access to both scrotal compartments. The affected testis is exposed first and the twisted spermatic cord is untwisted. The testis should be wrapped in a warm soaked swab if it fails to revascularize quickly and there is a question about its viability. Orchidectomy should not be undertaken unless the torsion is of long duration and the testis is obviously necrotic.

The viability of the testis may be checked by an intravenous injection of fluorescein and observation of the testis under an ultraviolet light. If the fluorescein perfuses the testis it is viable. At this point the testis must be fixed to prevent future torsion. A non-absorbable suture such as 3.0 nylon is used to fix the testis to the dartos muscle at two points, usually the inferior pole and midway on the lateral side of the testis. The unaffected testis should be fixed in a similar fashion, otherwise 10% will subsequently develop torsion. Prior to closure adequate attention to haemostasis with diathermy is necessary to prevent postoperative scrotal haematoma. Closure of the dartos is achieved by a continuous 3.0 chromic catgut suture. The scrotal skin is closed by a subcuticular or interrupted 3.0 chromic catgut. Non-absorbable sutures should not be used to close the scrotum. A scrotal support is prudent to minimize further the risk of postoperative scrotal haematoma. Non-absorbable sutures should not be used to anchor the testes to the dartos as torsion may recur when these sutures are absorbed.

4. Torsion affects 1 in 4000 males and is most common between the ages of 12 and 18 years. There have been reported cases of testicular torsion in neonates. The anatomical configuration predisposing to torsion is a high insertion of the tunica vaginalis on the spermatic cord combined with a narrow mesentery attached from the spermatic cord to the testis and epididymis which allows the testis to rotate like a clapper in a bell. Undescended testes are also at increased risk of torsion, especially if there is a tumour in the undescended testis.

5. The single most important determinant of a successful outcome, testicular salvage, is the duration of torsion prior to treatment. Correction within 4 h should preserve spermatogenesis and endocrine function in a previously healthy testis. Unfortunately, the mean time to presentation in adolescents, those most at risk of torsion, is often longer than 4 h, whilst the mean time to presentation in older men is usually shorter. Patients presenting with symptoms of intermittent torsion should have an urgent elective orchidopexy to prevent the risk of testicular loss due to acute torsion. Despite early intervention and apparent testicular salvage, many of these testes subsequently atrophy, presumably due to the effects of a sublethal ischaemic injury. Reported testicular salvage rates average 60%.

Tom Creagh

Case 27   Peripheral nerve injury

A 28-year-old professional guitarist was seen in casualty after accidentally cutting his right wrist when his hand shattered the glass pane as he was trying to open a window that had become jammed. On examination he had several superficial cuts of the right palm and a 1 cm laceration 4 cm proximal to the wrist on the ulnar border of the forearm. He was complaining of pain from his wounds, and numbness of the little finger was noted. Clinical examination suggested division of the ulnar nerve at the level of the wrist, which was subsequently confirmed on exploration.

Questions

1. How would you assess possible injury to the ulnar nerve?
2. Describe the surgical management of a divided ulnar nerve in the first 24 h.
3. Outline this patient's subsequent postoperative rehabilitation.
4. What are the postoperative complications following repair of a divided ulnar nerve?
5. Which factors influence eventual functional outcome following repair of a peripheral nerve?
6. How may recovery of peripheral nerve injury be assessed?

Answers

1. Lacerations to the hand and wrist by glass, even if apparently trivial, must raise the suspicion that nerves and tendons have been divided. Such injuries must be recognized and repaired promptly if a reasonable recovery is to be expected. Ask the patient about occupation, hand dominance, previous injuries and when he or she last had a tetanus vaccination.

   Whilst the wound should be inspected and the relationship to underlying structures noted, little will be gained from blindly probing within the laceration to define the extent of the damage – this will merely distress the patient and may result in further injury. Excessive bleeding can nearly always be controlled by simple elevation and pressure dressing – the use of clamps or haemostats is to be deprecated.

The sensory and motor function of the hand distal to the injury must be meticulously assessed, and if the original findings are equivocal re-examination later is often valuable. The ulnar nerve normally conveys sensory information from the ulnar $1\frac{1}{2}$ digits and corresponding part of the palm proximally to the level of the wrist, and supplies all the intrinsic muscles of the hand save the two most radial lumbricals and those of the thenar eminence. Inspection of the hand in a patient who has sustained an ulnar nerve lesion at the wrist will reveal a 'claw hand' (*main en griffe*), with hyperextension of the metacarpophalangeal joints of the ring and little fingers and flexion of the interphalangeal joints. With time, as the intrinsic muscles atrophy, the hypothenar eminence will become flattened and wasting of the interossei (notably in the first interosseous space between thumb and index finger) becomes obvious when the dorsum of the hand is inspected.

Motor function can be assessed by several tests which examine the intrinsic muscles – asking the patient to abduct the little finger against resistance has the advantage of allowing the examiner both to see and feel abductor digiti minimi contracting. Froment's test is also useful: the patient is asked to hold a card firmly between both extended thumbs and index fingers and prevent the examiner from dislodging it. Paralysis of adductor longus results in attempts to compensate by flexion of the interphalangeal joint via flexor pollicis longus. The difference between the normally extended and abnormally flexed thumb is obvious.

Due to sensory overlap the only area of sensation exclusive to the ulnar nerve is the little finger. Sensory loss should be evaluated by asking patients to close their eyes and tell the examiner whether they are being touched with a sharp or blunt object – total loss of sensation or poor discrimination should lead to the assumption that the nerve is damaged. Assessment of sweating should not be omitted as absence following nerve injury is often apparent before sensory loss can be convincingly demonstrated. Interruption of the sympathetic innervation produces vasodilatation (the ulnar digits look redder and may feel warmer than their more radial fellows), and whilst the absence of sweating is rarely obvious, the tactile adherence test is useful in detecting this valuable but more subtle sign. It may be performed by running a pen along the digits – the pen skids over the shiny dry surface of denervated skin (especially the pulp area), whilst there is a slight but appreciable drag when passing along a normal finger.

Radiographs taken in two planes, with soft-tissue views if indicated, must always be performed in injuries involving glass, which is nearly always radiopaque, although to a variable extent. This enables the location of shards which may otherwise be overlooked at operation and gives the surgeon valuable information on the number and distribution of the fragments preoperatively.

Always assess the integrity of any other structure that could conceivably have been injured – in practice, following glass injuries this means a formal assessment of all the motor, sensory and vascular components of the hand. All findings, both positive and negative, must be carefully recorded in the notes.

2. Primary repair (before a neuroma starts to form) of such injuries is preferable, which in practice is between 7 and 10 days following the insult, although ideally it should be effected within 24 h to maximize the chances of recovery. Good nerve repair requires excellent surgical technique and should only be performed by experienced surgeons, preferably in specialist units. Peripheral nerve injuries are often associated with either tendon or vessel damage, and such reconstructive surgery may take several hours – it is important that theatre staff are aware of this and that adequate theatre time is made available. For the comfort and compliance of the patient general anaesthesia is preferred. If this is not possible, a brachial plexus block may be employed. If these prerequisites cannot be fulfilled it is advisable to cover the wound with a suitable dressing, for example Betadine-soaked gauze, and wait the extra few hours rather than attempt a rushed repair by inexperienced staff with inadequate facilities.

The patient should be admitted and prepared for theatre. A note should be made as to when he or she last ate or drank, any appropriate investigations requested and the patient consented. The arm should be elevated preoperatively (a Bradford sling is ideal) to reduce the tissue swelling following injury. Once the patient is anaesthetized, anti-biotics, if indicated, should be administered and the limb then exsanguinated by elevation or application of an Esmarch bandage before application of a tourniquet to the upper arm, which is inflated to a pressure twice that of the patient's systolic pressure to ensure a bloodless field for surgery.

Nerve repair should be performed using magnification (either loupes or an operating microscope), bipolar dia-thermy, microsurgery instruments and suitable sutures – 8/0, 9/0 or 10/0 non-absorbable are all commonly used. The principle of nerve repair is accurate apposition of divided fascicles in a tension-free manner. The ulnar nerve has a small number of well-defined fascicles, and the varying sizes of these fascicles along with the vascular patterns on the epineurium provide valuable clues as to correct orien-tation during repair.

Peripheral nerves lie within a condensation of connective tissue, the epineurium, beneath which each fascicle is bounded by the tough perineurium. Individual axons with their investing Schwann cells lie within the delicate endo-neurial sheaths. The nerve derives its blood supply from a plexus of vessels running on and within the epineurium, which is fed in turn by branches from local arteries. Repair is effected by interrupted non-absorbable sutures – some advocate repair of individual fascicles before closure of the epineurium, but evidence is lacking that this is in any way superior.

The vascular supply may be occluded by undue long-itudinal tension, hence the importance of a tension-free repair, fortunately facilitated by the epineurial plexus which enables the nerve to be mobilized for some distance both proximally and distally without danger. Tendon and vessel repair, if necessary, should be performed before nerves are sutured as this also reduces tension across the nerve once mended. If a tension-free repair cannot be effected, better results are likely to result by use of an interposition graft using an expendable subcutaneous nerve such as the sural. Heavily contaminated wounds are a contraindication to nerve grafting but not to repair.

Once the ulnar nerve repair is complete, the skin should be closed and dressed with a non-adherent dressing under dry gauze. The forearm, wrist and hand should be wrapped with suitable padding and a dorsal backslab applied with the wrist flexed and in slight adduction to reduce tension across the restored nerve. The patient should be returned to the ward and the arm placed once more in a Bradford sling.

3. Gentle active finger exercises can commence on the day following operation under the supervision of a hand therapist. The sutures are removed at 2 weeks and the backslab and dressings discarded and replaced with a light-weight removable dorsal thermoplastic splint to keep the wrist partially flexed for a further 2–4 weeks. During this time vigorous activity of the fingers is encouraged, although the wrist should not be extended beyond neutral until splintage is no longer required. An alternative splintage is with dynamic 'lively' splints. The patient should be encouraged to use the hand as much as possible after splintage is discarded and qualified optimism may be expressed as to eventual restoration of function for up to 2 years following the injury.

4. Total failure of the repair may occur due to poor technique, inadequate postoperative splinting or a non-compliant patient. This will necessitate a secondary procedure with a consequent diminution of probable functional recovery. Loss of ulnar nerve function produces loss of metacarpophalangeal flexion and index finger abduction, resulting in an unstable pinch grip. Tendon transfers may improve hand function in such cases.

Following repair the nerve suture line may become adherent to adjacent structures, for example tendons (particularly when they too have been repaired), with consequent traction being applied to the nerve whenever the tendon moves. Treatment is by neurolysis. Painful neuromas may also occur and will require further operative intervention.

After a period of immobilization stiffness and weakness of the hand are inevitable. Recovery depends on the age and motivation of the patient, but fixed deformities may result in the older, poorly motivated individual. Supervised physiotherapy is required in all postoperative cases following injury to the hand or wrist, and patients must play an active part in both passive and active mobilization in between visits to outpatients.

Loss of sensation renders the affected part more liable to subsequent damage, especially burns, until recovery begins. The patient must be warned of this and advised on the prevention of such further injuries.

5. The most important factor governing outcome is the age of the patient. Following peripheral nerve repair, children can achieve a return of near normal sensory and motor function, but this is not the case in adults. This is probably a reflection of central nervous system plasticity in the young, allowing abnormal afferent sensory information to be processed better than in adults. Similarly, functional recovery is better following repair of a purely sensory or motor nerve when compared with a mixed nerve (such as the ulnar) which carries both types of axons.

   The severity of the injury affects final outcome – crushing injuries associated with significant soft-tissue damage and often complicated by subsequent infection carry a worse prognosis compared with clean lacerations. The level of injury is also important; the higher the lesion, the worse the outcome.

   Early diagnosis and intervention, surgical technique and effective rehabilitation are all areas where optimal care can enhance eventual outcome. It is important to repair associated vascular damage as studies have shown that prognosis following ulnar nerve repair is worse if a concomitant divided ulnar artery is neglected, presumably because this compromises the vascular plexus.

   Patients who subsequently develop neuromas, or who complain of symptoms of causalgia or paraesthesia, form a group whose outcome is likely to be poor; this is not necessarily so for patients with numbness or weakness which may continue to improve for some time.

6. Assessment of recovery is by return of motor and sensory function, which may continue for up to 2 years following surgical repair. It is important to consider recovery in the light of the patient's occupation and the extent to which the residual disability interferes with his or her activities of daily living. Axons regenerate at a rate of approximately 1 mm/day (following an initial delay of up to 1 month from the time of injury), and progress may be monitored clinically by lightly tapping over the course of the nerve – the patient will experience tingling or shooting pains over the distribution of the affected nerve when tapped over the tips of the regenerating axons; this is Tinel's test. More precise assessment

of the degree of nerve recovery can be obtained by electro-myelographic studies.

Further reading

Burke FD, McGrouther DA and Smith PJ. (1989) *The Principles of Hand Surgery*. Churchill Livingstone, Edinburgh

W. Burgoyne
Ciaran Healy

Case 28 Hepatitis

As a result of routine reporting and follow-up of cases of acute hepatitis B virus (HBV) infection in the UK, three cases were found to have had major surgery by the same surgeon in the previous 8 months. With the surgeon's cooperation, his blood was tested for HBV markers with the following results: hepatitis B surface antigen (HBsAg) positive, HBeAg positive, anti HBc antibody-positive. The surgeon was in good health, his liver function tests were normal and he had no history of acute hepatitis.

Questions

1. What advice should be given to the surgeon?
2. What can be done to investigate the outbreak?
3. How significant is the risk of transmission of HBV from health care workers to their patients?
4. Describe the nature of hepatitis B vaccines and the significance of follow-up testing for immunity.

Answers

1. The surgeon was found to be a carrier of hepatitis B virus by a positive result in the screening test for HBsAg. The test for e antigen (HBeAg) provides a marker for potential infectivity. Individuals are normally HBeAg-positive during the acute phase of the illness and approximately 5% of adults infected in Europe and North America progress to the carrier state. If individuals remain HBeAg-positive, they are likely to have persistence of infectious virus in their blood, abnormal liver function and the danger of developing chronic liver disease and cirrhosis and they have an increased risk of hepatocellular carcinoma. There is a risk of transmission to sexual partners and others by blood transfer and women are likely to transmit to their babies during labour. These risks from horizontal transmission can be removed if the close contacts, including neonates, are successfully immunized.

The first advice to the surgeon must be to stop operating and to avoid any procedures which may expose patients to his blood. As a result of continuing reports of transmission of hepatitis B virus from infected health care workers to their patients during the course of surgical and dental procedures, new guidelines were introduced by the health departments in the UK in August 1993. All health care workers engaged in exposure-prone procedures should be immunized against hepatitis B. Exposure-prone procedures are defined as follows: 'Those procedures where there is a risk that injury to the health care worker may result in the exposure of the patient's open tissues to the blood of the worker. These procedures include those where the worker's gloved hand may be in contact with sharp instruments, needle tips or sharp tissues (spicules of bone or teeth) inside a patient's open body cavity, wound or confined anatomical space where the hands or finger tips may not be completely visible at all times'.

Non-responders to the vaccine should be investigated to ensure that they are not hepatitis B carriers and if their lack of response results from vaccine failure they should be offered specific immunonglobulin (HBIg) in the event of inoculation injury. HBeAg-positive health care workers should not participate in exposure-prone invasive procedures. This may obviously have major career implications as effectively a surgeon may need to move to another branch of medicine and this may necessitate a programme of retraining.

Note: These guidelines have been adopted in the UK and do not necessarily apply to other countries.

The surgeon should be referred for a specialist opinion from a hepatologist. Further assessment of his liver function, including, if appropriate, liver biopsy, may lead to the possibility of treatment with interferon-alpha. If response to treatment is successful, with the disappearance of HBeAg from the circulation and the appearance of antibodies to HBeAg, there is the possibility that the surgeon may be able to return to operative surgery.

2. In the UK, the Director of Public Health may decide, in collaboration with the Department of Health Advisory Panel for Health Care Workers Infected with Bloodborne Viruses, to conduct a retrospective study of other patients who had undergone surgery by the infected surgeon. This is

obviously a major step to take as notification of patients long after they had recovered from their operations is likely to generate anxiety. As asymptomatic attacks of hepatitis B are common, a study of this type would normally involve counselling and testing of a blood sample from each patient for HBsAg.

Before embarking on such a study it may be sensible to confirm that there has indeed been occupational transmission of hepatitis B virus and that the three cases occurring after surgery in these patients did not result from some other route of transmission. Identity between the virus from the surgeon and those from his patients can be confirmed by DNA sequencing of the virus present in blood samples. This process of genetic fingerprinting is available in specialized virology units.

3. It has been recognized for many years that hepatitis B-infected health care workers can transmit the virus to their patients during the course of surgical or dental procedures. In the period 1975–1990, 12 outbreaks of HBV infection associated with infected surgical staff (11 surgeons and one perfusion technician) were reported in England, Wales and Northern Ireland, and these were known to have resulted in transmission to 95 patients. In all but one of these outbreaks the source health care worker was HBeAg-positive; information on the infectivity status of the remaining surgeon is unavailable.

   Following the appearance in 1989 of clinical hepatitis in three patients undergoing gynaecological surgery in London, the gynaecologist concerned was found to be an HBeAg-positive carrier of hepatitis B. Retrospective testing of a further 247 of his patients revealed that 22 had markers of recent or current hepatitis B and five were symptomatic. The transmission rates recorded for the highest-risk procedures were 10/42 (23.8%) for hysterectomy and 10/51 (19.5%) for caesarean section. Reported rates for hepatitis B transmission in other types of surgical and dental procedures where the main operator was a carrier of the virus are as given in Table 28.1.

4. Two types of vaccine have been developed for hepatitis B immunization. Both are effective in preventing infection with the development of long-term antibody and both are of acceptably low toxicity.

Table 28.1 Hepatitis B transmission in procedures where the main operator is a carrier of the virus

Procedure	Number	Percentage
Cardiac surgery	5/69	7.2%
Coronary artery bypass	17/231	7.3%
Orthopaedic surgery	49/1532	3.2%
Oral surgery	6/395	1.5%
	52/570	9.1%
	52/511	10.2%
General dentistry	23/711	3.2%

(a) *Plasma-derived vaccine:* The first hepatitis B vaccine to be produced was obtained by plasmapheresis of blood donors found to be carriers of hepatitis B. By a long and carefully controlled extraction and inactivation process, particles of HBsAg were extracted from their plasma and this natural product was formulated into the vaccine preparation.

(b) *Genetically engineered vaccines:* With the development of recombinant DNA vaccines it has become possible to insert the gene encoding HBsAg into a variety of vector systems. By incorporation of the gene into a yeast vector it is possible, by a process of fermentation, to produce large quantities of HBsAg for production of vaccines. Obviously this product, derived from a synthetic gene sequence, is guaranteed to be free from contamination with any other viral or human components. These vaccines are currently in routine use.

Every vaccination procedure has a failure rate and hepatitis B immunization is no exception. In the most responsive groups (i.e. young women) there may be a failure rate, after a full course of vaccine, of 5%. The failure rate is higher in men and increases with advancing age. Immunocompromised individuals are generally less likely than those with normal immunity to respond to hepatitis B vaccines. The acknowledged failure rate of the vaccine is one reason for the need to test for immunity after a full course of injections. Administration of a fourth dose of vaccine often produces a response when the standard course of three injections has failed. In addition, health care workers at risk of infection need to know the magnitude of their response to determine the strength of their protection and to predict the need for future booster doses. An antibody level of <10 miu/ml indicates a failure to respond. Between 10 and 100 miu/ml is a weak response and one would normally recommend boosting with a fourth dose of vaccine. Over 100 miu/ml is a good response and should not require boosting for 3–5 years.

Further reading

Jeffries DJ. (1995) Viral hazards to and from health care workers. *Journal of Hospital Infection* **30**(suppl): 140–155

Donald J. Jeffries

Case 29   Infected foreskin: the place of medical circumcision

A 3-year-old, healthy boy is referred to the urology clinic for recurrent foreskin infections associated with occasional discomfort during micturition. Physical examination demonstrates normal genitalia and a mildly inflamed foreskin which is partially retractable.

Questions

1. What are the therapeutic options available to help this boy?
2. What are the possible complications of circumcision?
3. What are the medical indications of circumcision?
4. What are the contraindications of circumcision?

Answers

1. There are three principal therapeutic approaches for recurrent foreskin infections:
   (a) The medical treatment should be the first choice. *Oral antibiotics are not necessary* since it is a local problem which requires a local treatment. Application (or penile baths) of a solution of *aqueous* chlorhexidine on the foreskin twice a day for a few days stops local infection and inflammation in most cases. Alternatively, an application of chloramphenicol ointment (used by ophthalmologists) on the foreskin may also help.
      If this first-line treatment does not solve the problem, other therapeutic options should be considered.
   (b) Circumcision is the traditional treatment of recurrent foreskin infections. It is a radical and somewhat unpleasant procedure, often performed by inexperienced surgeons, and consequently bears a significant risk of complications of various severity. However, it sorts out the local symptoms in all cases and remains a standard treatment in Northern Europe and the USA. It is said that circumcision may prevent penile cancers and cervical

cancer in the partner and reduce the incidence of sexually transmitted diseases.

(c) Alternatively, a simple division of preputial adhesions (foreskin stretch) or a preputial plasty (widening of the foreskin) also gives excellent results and these are nontraumatic procedures with almost no complication. These two procedures keep the foreskin intact and this has some medical advantages (protection of the glans mucosa and urethral meatus), and some cultural advantages, especially in continental Europe where circumcision is not a well-accepted procedure.

2. The complications of circumcision are common:

(a) Immediate complications:

(i) Penile bruising and oedema are frequent and can easily be resolved by penile baths with an *aqueous* solution of chlorhexidine.

(ii) Intraoperative and postoperative bleeding and local infection can be severe and may occasionally require a second procedure.

(iii) Penile injuries, including glans amputation, are also reported, especially with the plasty-bell technique or with religious circumcisions.

(b) Long-term complications are less reported although not rare:

(i) Bad cosmetic results are common when too much or not enough penile skin has been excised. Skin bridges are the result of inappropriate mucosal excision. Secondary procedures are then often required.

(ii) Urethrocutaneous fistula, often due to an inconsiderate use of diathermy, is a severe complication requiring a secondary urethroplasty.

(iii) Meatal stenosis is the most common long-term complication of circumcision and is revealed either by a penile or abdominal pain at initiation of micturition, or a fine stream with high pressure forcing the child to step back or to sit on the toilet. The child's mother often describes a considerable amount of urine spillage around the toilet bowl after each micturition. Clinical examination shows a pin-hole meatus bridged by a filmy membrane, whereas the rest of the glans mucosa remains normal (no balanitis xerotica obliterans). This complication is not always recognized and requires a meatotomy.

(iv) Sexual discomfort is more and more reported and some surgeons are now proposing uncircumcision procedures for these patients.

3. The American Academy of Pediatrics has stated that 'there is no absolute medical indication for routine circumcision in the newborn'. The vast majority of circumcisions are therefore performed for religious, cultural or personal reasons.
   The medical indications remain:
   (a) Scarred irretractable foreskin (or secondary phimosis).
   (b) Recurrent foreskin infections in diabetic patients.
   (c) The true phimosis or primary phimosis (impossible to retract the foreskin due to a congenital tight preputial opening) can also be treated by a preputial plasty, which is less invasive and keeps the foreskin almost intact.
   (d) Infants under 1 year old with recurrent urinary tract infections and vesicoureteric reflux may benefit from circumcision, although it has not been scientifically proven yet.

4. The contraindications of circumcision:
   (a) Hypospadias where the preputial hood is often used for the urethroplasty.
   (b) Clotting disorders (such as haemophilia) are a relative contraindication.
   (c) Buried penis, which requires specific surgical operations but not circumcision.

Further reading

Bigelow J. (1992) *The Joy of Uncircumcising! Restore your Birthright and Maximize Sexual Pleasure*. Hourglass, Aptos

Cuckow PM, Rix G and Mouriquand PDE. (1994) Preputial plasty: a good alternative to circumcision. *Journal of Pediatric Surgery* **29:** 561–563

Goodwin WE (1990) Uncircumcision: a technique for plastic reconstruction of a prepuce after circumcision. *Journal of Urology* **144:** 1203–1205

Gordon A and Collin J. (1993) Save the normal foreskin. *British Medical Journal* **306:** 1–2

Kaplan GW. (1988) Newborn circumcision: controversy revisited. *Dialysis and Pediatric Urology* **11:** 1–8

Kunin SA. (1994) Circumcision in newborns: not why, but how. *Dialysis and Pediatric Urology* **17:** 1–8

Martinowitz U, Varon D, Bar-Maor A, Brenner B, Leibovitch I and Heim M. (1992) Circumcision in hemophilia: the use of fibrin glue for local hemostasis. *Journal of Urology* **148:** 855–857

Patel H. (1966) The problem of routine circumcision. *Canadian Medical Association Journal* **95:** 576–581

Persad R, Sharma S, McTavish J and Mouriquand PDE. (1995) Clinical presentation and pathophysiology of meatal stenosis following circumcision. *British Journal of Urology* **75:** 91–93

Redman JF. (1900) Circumcision revision in prepubertal boys: analysis of a 2-year experience and description of a technique. *Journal of Urology* **153:** 180–182

Roberts JA. (1986) Does circumcision prevent urinary tract infection? *Journal of Urology* **135:** 991–992

Williams N, Chell J and Kapila L. (1993) Why are children referred for circumcision? *British Medical Journal* **306:** 28

Wiswell TE and Roscelli JD. (1986) Corroborative evidence for the decreased incidence of urinary tract infections in circumcised male infants. *Pediatrics* **78:** 96–99

Woodside JR. (1980) Circumcision disasters. *Pediatrics* **65:** 1053–1054

Multiple choice questions

1. **Circumcision:**
   (a) Circumcision at birth is recommended to prevent penile carcinoma.
   (b) Circumcision remains the only treatment of recurrent foreskin infections.
   (c) Complications following circumcision are rare.
   (d) Medical indications of circumcision are rare.

d is the correct answer.

2. **Foreskin infections:**
   (a) Preputial plasty is a safe alternative to circumcision.
   (b) Local antiseptic treatment should be the first option in boys with recurrent foreskin infections.
   (c) Oral antibiotic is the treatment of choice of recurrent foreskin infections.
   (d) Recurrent foreskin infections only occur in diabetic patients.

a and b are the correct answers.

3. **Circumcision:**
   (a) Diabetes is a contraindication of circumcision.
   (b) Hypospadias is a contraindication of circumcision.
   (c) Haemophilia is an absolute contraindication of circumcision.
   (d) Meatal stenosis is the most common long-term complication of circumcision.

b and d are correct.

Y. Mor
P.D.E. Mouriquand

Case 30   Acute pain management

A 63-year-old man had undergone a routine laparotomy and anterior resection 24 h ago. The patient had an epidural catheter in place, and an infusion was given via the epidural for the first 12 h. The pain relief had become less effective over the previous 6 h and the pain team examined the patient and found that the epidural catheter had been misplaced. The patient was then given a patient-controlled analgesia (PCA) machine. The patient has become drowsy over the last hour and has a respiratory rate of 9 breaths/min. He is not in pain, and his oxygen saturation is 97%. He is receiving 28% oxygen from a Hudson mask. The nurses are concerned about his state of consciousness.

Questions

1. What is the likely aetiology?
2. What is the significance of the epidural infusion?
3. What is the management of this patient?
4. What is the implication of the oxygen saturation?

Answers

1. The likely aetiology in this case is a degree of respiratory depression due to an overdose of opioid drugs, but other causes of reduced consciousness should be considered and eliminated before this diagnosis is made. PCA is a system whereby analgesic drugs are self-administered. This includes self-medication with oral analgesic drugs, but the term is usually used in the context of a system designed to give intravenous opiate drugs on demand. There are a number of machines on the market, but they have several features in common. They have a bolus dosing system, a lock-out time which prevents patients from giving themselves boluses at less than the time interval, and they have an antisyphon device for preventing a whole syringe of opiate being drawn into an intravenous infusion. Expensive electronic devices and cheaper, simple, mechanical devices are available.

The drug used can be varied, but commonly the boluses are either morphine 1 or 2 mg, or pethidine 10 mg. Lock-out times are a minimum of 5 min, but may be longer where higher bolus doses are used. The simple devices usually have a fixed lock-out time, but can be filled with solutions of different strength to give different bolus sizes. The more complex and expensive electronic devices can alter both. The patient is given a handpiece with a sensor which when pressed delivers a bolus. Subsequent pressing will not produce a bolus until the lock-out time is reached. Sophisticated devices will record the dose/demand ratio which can be useful in assessing the appropriateness of the bolus size.

The PCA system is inherently safe because the patient will administer the drug as required, and if patients inadvertently give themselves sufficient opiate to become drowsy, they will be unable to press the button until this effect has worn off. The danger arises when opiates are additionally given by another route.

2. The epidural infusion given before the PCA system was started is of particular importance in this case: infusions are in common use after major abdominal surgery, as they confer benefits beyond analgesia in terms of surgical outcome. The infusion regimens commonly comprise a mixture of local anaesthetics, usually bupivicaine, and an opiate, diamorphine or fentanyl. It is important to check whether opiates were used in the infusion because opiates given into the epidural space can cause side-effects for as long as 12 h after the termination of the infusion. This is due to diffusion of the opiate drug through the dura into the cerebrospinal fluid (CSF). Lipid-soluble opiates are largely bound to the dorsal horn of the spinal cord. Some less lipid-soluble opiates, notably morphine, but any of the drugs can produce this, remain in the CSF and are carried upwards with the circulation of CSF, eventually reaching the respiratory centre and causing late respiratory depression. If this were the case then the diagnosis of respiratory depression due to a combination of epidural and PCA opiate becomes more likely. It is important to establish whether opiates have been inadvertently given by other routes, such as intramuscularly or subcutaneously, in addition to the PCA.

3. The optimal management of this patient requires him to be prevented from developing severe respiratory depression, whilst at the same time attempting to give him analgesia.

The assessment of respiratory depression cannot be made on the respiratory rate alone, nor is it reasonable to assume that because he has an acceptable oxygen saturation there is no cause for concern. Oxygen saturation will be maintained during very slow breathing if the patient is breathing a high inspired oxygen. In this case the patient is breathing 28% oxygen, so the saturation is not a guide to the degree of respiratory depression. In this situation the danger arises from the rise in partial pressure of carbon dioxide in the blood, which may be considerable, the results of which are acidosis, arrhythmias and narcosis. Arterial carbon dioxide can be established from a blood-gas sample, which should be taken if the patient is deeply comatose. In this case the patient is drowsy but rousable, the respiratory rate is low, opiates have been given, and their effects can be reversed by the use of the μ-receptor antagonist drug naloxone (0.4 mg i.v.). There are disadvantages to giving naloxone in this context, as it will also reverse the analgesic effect of the opiate. Therefore if the situation will permit, the patient should be closely observed by the nursing staff, the PCA removed from his reach, but not taken down, and his respiratory rate recorded; if it drops further then naloxone can be given in 0.1 mg increments to minimize the amount used. Naloxone has a short half-life, and the dosage may need to be repeated in 20 min to maintain a respiratory rate above 8 breaths/min. As long as no more opiates are administered until the patient is alert and breathing at greater than 10 breaths/min, observation of an increasing respiratory rate is the ideal outcome. If the PCA remains attached to the drip but is out of the patient's reach until he is rousable, then it can be reintroduced when required.

4. This case illustrates the false sense of security that can be engendered by the use of pulse oximetry monitoring in patients who are receiving additional oxygen. It is now common practice to give postoperative patients who are receiving opiates oxygen via a mask. This is based on research that shows that postoperative patients receiving opiates will have periods of desaturation of their haemoglobin during the night on the first 3 postoperative nights. The significance of these episodes of desaturation is not clear but they can hardly be considered as desirable, hence the increased use of oxygen. The important aspect of this is that, despite normal oxygen saturation, the patient's

respiration can become depressed, especially if opiates are given by more than one route. That respiratory depression should be treated if necessary with naloxone, but this will result in a patient in pain. If nursing staff are able to observe the patient for further respiratory depression closely then natural recovery may avoid the use of naloxone.

Further reading

Harmer M, Rosen M and Vickers MD (eds) (1985) *Patient Controlled Analgesia.* Blackwell Scientific Publications, Oxford

The Royal College of Surgeons of England, College of Anaesthetists (1990) *Commission on the Provision of Surgical Services. Report of the Working Party on Pain after Surgery.*

Lesley Bromley

Case 31 Ulcerative colitis

A 24-year-old Caucasian man was referred by the gastroenterologists, having been admitted under their care from outpatients with severe bloody diarrhoea, abdominal pain and lethargy. He had been diagnosed as having ulcerative colitis 3 years previously, and had been admitted briefly in 1992 for medical treatment. His symptoms were normally controlled with mesalazine 400 mg t.d.s. and azathioprine but in the last 8 weeks he had experienced bloody diarrhoea, with his bowels open approximately 30 times each 24 h. Over the last year he had lost 15 kg, and his current weight was 57 kg. On examination, the patient was found to be apyrexial, have a pulse rate of 110 beats/min and a blood pressure of 100/55 mmHg. Abdominal examination revealed a soft distended abdomen with tenderness but no guarding. He had been investigated by the gastroenterologists and had received a 2 u blood transfusion. Intravenous steroids, and subsequently intravenous cyclosporin, had been given. Having failed to respond to medical treatment, he was referred for a surgical opinion.

Questions

1. How would you investigate this patient on admission?
2. Describe the medical treatment of acute ulcerative colitis.
3. What are the possible local complications of ulcerative colitis?
4. What are the surgical options in the management of ulcerative colitis?
5. What extraintestinal problems occur with ulcerative colitis?

Answers

1. Sigmoidoscopy should be performed without preparation to assess the presence and severity of the inflammation. In mild colitis, there will be loss of vascular pattern, and the mucosa appears hyperaemic and oedematous. With more severe inflammation, the mucosa becomes granular with

contact haemorrhage and eventually ulcerated. Pseudo-polyp formation from previous attacks may be evident. If the diagnosis has not already been established then a rectal biopsy should be performed unless there is fulminating colitis. Stool specimens should be cultured to look for *Salmonella, Shigella, Campylobacter* species and to exclude *Clostridium difficile*, and the microbiologist should be informed of these possibilities. In a new presentation fresh stool specimens should be examined for amoebiasis. Laboratory investigations should include a full blood count, urea and electrolytes, erythrocyte sedimentation rate (ESR), C-reactive protein and liver function tests. Many patients develop a hypochromic microcytic anaemia with iron deficiency. In active disease there is often a leukocytosis, with an eosinophilia and thrombocytosis. Hypokalaemia, hypoalbuminaemia and an elevated aspartate aminotransferase or alkaline phosphatase also occur.

A plain supine abdominal X-ray should be performed in all patients with a severe attack. It is important to distinguish between toxic megacolon and acute severe colitis. Acute toxic dilatation is inferred if the diameter of the colon in any part is greater than 5.5 cm with loss of normal haustra. In severe cases, mucosal islands may be seen. The presence of intramural air suggests imminent perforation. Free air may be seen on a plain abdominal radiograph. The plain film will enable some assessment of the extent of disease. Mucosal oedema and ulceration may be apparent, and the affected colon may be widened and distended with air. Faecal residue is rarely present in an inflamed segment. More information can be gained from an unprepared instant enema using water-soluble contrast, although this is contraindicated in toxic megacolon.

2. Attacks of ulcerative colitis may be defined as:
   (a) Severe, with passage of more than six stools daily with blood and systemic disturbance such as fever, tachycardia, anaemia or an ESR ≥ 30 mm/h.
   (b) Mild with four or fewer stools per day with little or no blood, no systemic disturbance and a normal ESR.
   (c) Moderate, which includes the remaining patients.

Mild to moderate attacks can be managed with oral prednisolone 20–40 mg combined with sulphasalazine and steroid enemas. The steroids should be tailed down to 20 mg after 1 week. Remission is maintained using sulphasalazine, mesalazine or olsalazine. Patients with severe attacks should be admitted, and may require correction of electrolyte and fluid loss, and transfusion for anaemia. Intravenous steroids, for example prednisolone 60 mg or hydrocortisone 400 mg/d and hydrocortisone enemas 100 mg twice a day, may be given. Regular review of the patient's clinical condition and daily plain abdominal radiographs may be required in the first few days. The nutritional status of the patient should be assessed and may require improvement with intravenous nutrition. Those who respond well (70%) should continue on oral steroids and sulphasalazine. Urgent colectomy should be considered in those failing to respond. Some clinicians have used intravenous cyclosporin A in those who do not respond, and there is some evidence that this can be effective in the acute attack but it may not change the colectomy rate in the intermediate term.

3. Perforation occurs in those with severe disease and is more common during the first attack. Although the most dangerous of complications, early surgical treatment of toxic dilatation in the last 20 years has reduced the risk. Corticosteroids may mask the symptoms but there is no evidence that steroid therapy predisposes to perforation. Treatment is by emergency colectomy with ileostomy and peritoneal lavage. Mortality still approaches 50%.

Toxic dilatation presents with general deterioration, tachycardia and abdominal distension. It occurs more commonly in those with total colitis during their first attack and is a precursor to perforation. Patients require fluid and electrolyte replacement and intravenous steroids. Although 30% respond to medical management, the ultimate outcome is often colectomy in these patients. Most patients will require urgent colectomy after correction of the metabolic disturbances.

A few patients with colitis suffer major haemorrhage. When it occurs it often arises from rectal ulceration and urgent colectomy alone in such cases may therefore not be sufficient and part of the rectum may also require removal. Benign stricture formation may rarely occur in long-standing disease, and pseudopolyps are commonly found after recurrent attacks. These may be large but have no malignant potential. Patients with long-standing extensive ulcerative colitis have a significantly greater risk of developing colorectal cancer. The risk starts to increase 10 years after diagnosis and progresses at a cumulative rate of 1% per year thereafter.

4. When emergency surgery for acute severe ulcerative colitis is required, colectomy and ileostomy is most commonly performed. For those likely to undergo either restorative proctocolectomy or ileorectal anastomosis at a later stage, the rectum should be divided at or above the pelvic brim, and brought out as a mucous fistula or closed close to the abdominal wall. The decision to close the rectal stump will depend on the surgeon's assessment of the state of the patient and the condition of the bowel.

Indications for elective surgery are failed medical treatment, malignant (or dysplastic) change and growth retardation in a child. In these situations a colectomy is needed in all cases but the surgical choice lies between preserving the rectum and anus; preserving the anus only or excising both rectum and anus. Thus the options include:

(a) Proctocolectomy with ileostomy, which may be performed in those patients in whom there is no possibility of later restorative surgery. In such patients, in the absence of malignancy, an intersphincteric dissection is preferred.

(b) Colectomy with ileorectal anastomosis should be considered if there is minimal inflammation in the rectum, and the patient is likely to comply with close sigmoidoscopic follows-up, if the rectum is not markedly diseased. However, a significant number of patients have a poor functional result and later require completion proctectomy. In addition, rectal carcinoma occurs in approximately 15% of patients after 25 years, often in an advanced stage. Nevertheless, the operation gives a satisfactory long-term result in around 50% of patients.

(c) Restorative proctocolectomy with ileoanal anastomosis removes all affected bowel whilst preserving the anal sphincter mechanism, thus avoiding a permanent stoma. This should be performed electively, not in the acute situation. More than half the patients have previously had an emergency colectomy. A covering loop ileostomy is usually formed, although the need for the stoma and the advisability of a mucosectomy to excise the anal transitional zone are still debated.

(d) A Koch continent ileostomy may be offered to selected patients who have previously had a proctectomy and are keen to avoid conventional ileostomy. It allows the majority of patients to manage without an ileostomy bag, but revisional surgery is needed in 10–40% of patients. It can be performed as a first-stage procedure or when restorative procedures have been unsuccessful.

5. Skin: erythema nodosum and pyoderma gangrenosum occur in association with ulcerative colitis. Erythema nodosum more commonly affects women and presents typically as tender red nodules over the anterior aspect of the lower limbs, but may affect the arms or hands. The lesions may ulcerate, but more commonly leave a light brown discoloration. Unlike pyoderma, development of nodules coincides with disease activity. Pyoderma gangrenosum presents as a painful necrotic ulcer and, although it occurs elsewhere, it typically affects the lower limb. In some patients pyoderma resolves after colectomy.

A range of eye problems has been described in association with ulcerative colitis. Uveitis is the most common, being reported in approximately 4% of patients. Other eye conditions include episcleritis and keratoconjunctivitis. Symptomatic patients complain of blurred vision, eye pain, photophobia and headache and respond to treatment with local or systemic steroids.

Liver function can be abnormal in ulcerative colitis for a number of reasons. These range from minor biochemical changes to cirrhosis. Changes affecting the biliary tree, such as pericholangitis, primary sclerosing cholangitis, gallstones and biliary tract carcinoma may occur. Parenchymal disease may include fatty change, chronic active hepatitis or cirrhosis. Iatrogenic causes of altered liver function include drug therapy and total parenteral nutrition.

Arthritis may complicate ulcerative colitis, and can be activity-related or independent of the state of the disease. Activity-related or enteropathic arthritis involves synovial inflammation which usually affects the large joints of the lower limbs, but any joint may be involved. Treatments include non-steroidal anti-inflammatory drugs or Salazopyrin. Colectomy in cases of fulminating colitis may result in remission of arthritis. Ankylosing spondylitis may be asymptomatic and is not related to the severity of the colitis. A third of patients with colitis-associated ankylosing spondylitis are human leukocyte antigen (HLA)-B27-positive; 95% of patients with sporadic ankylosing spondylitis are

HLA-B27-positive. Non-steroidal anti-inflammatory drugs and exercise are used to treat symptomatic patients.

Further reading

Mortensen NJ, Nicholls RJ, Northover JMA and Williams NS. (1992) The colon, rectum and anus. In: Burnand KG and Young AE (eds) *The New Aird's Companion in Surgical Studies*. Churchill Livingstone, Edinburgh, pp. 1021–1096

Christopher T.M. Speakman
Humphrey Scott
R. John Nicholls

Case 32 Postoperative pneumonia

A 76-year-old woman is admitted to the surgical ward with an acute abdomen. She gave a history of passing blood per rectum a few weeks before admission, and had noted abdominal distension and constipation for 3 days. The patient gave a past history of mild hypertension and her only medication was Moduretic once daily. She was a non-smoker and drank alcohol occasionally. On examination her pulse was 92 beats/min, sinus rhythm, and the blood pressure 130/70 mmHg. The central venous pressure was not elevated and the heart clinically mildly enlarged with the apex beat displaced laterally 2 cm. Examination of the heart and chest were normal apart from a few fine crepitations at the base of the right lung. Abdominal examination revealed general tenderness, with guarding and pain on palpation in the left iliac fossa.

The abdominal X-ray was consistent with large-bowel obstruction and at laparotomy a Hartmann's procedure was performed for extensive sigmoid diverticular disease. Postoperatively she became rather confused with a pyrexia (38.2°C), and percussion was dull at the base of the right lung.

Questions

1. What is the most likely diagnosis?
2. Discuss the investigations you would perform to confirm the diagnosis.
3. What treatment would you initiate?

Answers

1. The differential diagnosis is of either a chest infection or pulmonary embolism. As the patient had been unwell prior to admission to hospital, she was clearly exposed to the risk of deep venous thrombosis. Also, elderly patients who are immobile are at greater risk of pneumonia, which is exacerbated in this case by the shallow breathing as a result of the abdominal surgery. Your initial investigations should include

a full blood count (to assess the haemoglobin and white cell count, although the latter will be elevated as a result of the diverticular disease and surgery), electrolytes and arterial blood gases. A chest X-ray should be compared to the preoperative film, making due allowance for the fact that this film will be an anteroposterior film taken using portable equipment. Supplemental oxygen should be given (see below), a sputum sample obtained if possible (without delaying therapy) and the antibiotics changed to include a broad-spectrum penicillin or erythromycin if the patient is allergic to penicillins (via a large vein to reduce the risk of phlebitis).

2. In many elderly patients, confusion may be the only sign of a postoperative pneumonia, and care must be taken to distinguish between the chest infection as a cause of hypoxia and pulmonary embolism and/or heart failure. This may not be easy, but must be done, as prescribing inappropriate treatment such as administering diuretics to a vasodilated patient with a pyrexia secondary to pneumonia will reduce cardiac output with dire consequences.

The chest X-ray may be unremarkable, particularly if the patient has a history of chronic bronchitis and has retained mucus in the bronchi postoperatively. The dull percussion note in the chest indicates the presence of consolidation or a pleural effusion or both. The clinical and radiographic features of pneumonia may be secondary to atelectasis (collapse of alveoli due to postoperative hypoventilation induced by the painful abdominal wound) or due to pooled secretions in more elderly and immobile patients. Physiotherapy should be performed regularly to ensure expectoration of mucus and help reduce the risk of secondary or superimposed infection.

The electrolytes may have been somewhat deranged on admission as patients receiving Moduretic tend to have a degree of hyponatraemia, and this will be compounded by intrathoracic pathology (including pneumonia) which produces an increase in antidiuretic hormone production and haemodilution. A more common cause of hyponatraemia however is excessive administration of dextrose in the postoperative period.

The arterial blood-gas results are important in reaching your diagnosis and in determining the most appropriate therapy. The results should be interpreted in the light of whether there was any previous history of lung disease as patients with chronic obstructive lung disease (who are more susceptible to postoperative chest infections) will have been relatively hypoxic before admission and will also have an increased tendency to carbon dioxide retention. In such patients, the arterial gases must be repeated after initiating supplemental oxygen, as higher concentrations of inspired oxygen may relieve the hypoxia but remove the respiratory drive as the carbon dioxide rises. Hypoxia with a low carbon dioxide level and no antecedent history of chest disease should alert you to pulmonary embolism, especially if the chest X-ray is normal. An ECG and cardiac enzymes should also be recorded, although the latter may be abnormal due to muscle division during surgery. Isoenzyme analysis (such as creatine kinase [CK-MB]) may be helpful in such situations.

3. In this patient the chest X-ray reveals extensive right lower-zone consolidation with a small overlying pleural effusion. The most common pathogens are the pneumococcus and *Haemophilus* species, although others may have to be considered, including *Staphylococcus aureus*, *Klebsiella*, *Legionella* and Gram-negative organisms (particularly if there is any suggestion of aspiration). The antibiotic regimen should be determined by considering whether the infection was acquired before admission or was acquired in hospital. This may of course be impossible to say, but the latter should be treated with cefuroxime and gentamicin (and perhaps erythromycin) intravenously. Aspiration should be treated with benzylpenicillin, metronidazole and gentamicin, the last according to a nomogram with careful monitoring of drug levels to reduce the risk of nephropathy and ototoxicity. In patients with serious infection, early discussion with the hospital microbiologist is important as hospital antibiotic policies must be followed to reduce the risk from resistant organisms, or from *Clostridium difficile*, which may follow extensive use of broad-spectrum antibiotics, including the cephalosporins. Careful attention must be paid to ensure satisfactory ventilation (by regular assessment of the arterial blood gases) and fluid balance. Measurement of the central venous pressure by a centrally placed catheter should be considered early in the course of a significant postoperative pneumonia to ensure optimum hydration and adequate replacement of insensible losses.

Further reading

British Thoracic Society (1993) Guidelines for the management of community acquired pneumonia in adults admitted to hospital. *British Journal of Hospital Medicine* **49:** 346–350

Hope RA and Longmore JM (eds) (1993) *Oxford Handbook of Clinical Medicine*, 3rd edn. Oxford University Press, Oxford

Drugs used in the treatment of infection: current edition of the *British National Formulary* (British Medical Association/Royal Pharmaceutical Society of Great Britain, London) which should be used in conjunction with the hospital antibiotic policy regarding antibiotic choice and dosage

D.P. Dutka

Case 33   Oesophageal carcinoma

A 38-year-old female presented with a history of dysphagia for solids and 6.5 kg (1 stone) weight loss. This had been progressive for 9 weeks but she had had several previous episodes of dysphagia. She smoked 10 cigarettes a day and was a nondrinker. In her past medical history she had a partial gastrectomy for a bleeding gastric ulcer 20 years previously. She had a history of severe reflux oesophagitis for 15 years with a stricture which had required dilatation elsewhere. Examination was grossly normal.

Questions

1. What is your differential diagnosis? What is the most likely diagnosis?
2. What is the epidemiology of this problem?
3. Are there any known risk factors for this condition?
4. Is there any role for adjuvant or neoadjuvant therapy?
5. What is her prognosis?

Answers

1. Once again, the history of dysphagia and weight loss suggests oesophageal carcinoma. In this case the long history of reflux suggests Barrett's oesophagus and the symptoms may be explained by a stricture or severe oesophagitis. Severe oesophagitis in turn may be associated with a motility disorder. Achalasia should be considered but the rapid onset of severe dysphagia is against it. Diverticula of the oesophagus are less common in this age group.

    Two points in her history add further weight to the suspicion of carcinoma, particularly adenocarcinoma. There is an association between previous gastric surgery and oesophageal adenocarcinoma. The long reflux history suggests Barrett's oesophagus and this is a potentially premalignant lesion, associated with an increased risk of adenocarcinoma of about 1 in 150 patient-years.

2. There is enormous variation in the incidence of oesophageal cancer throughout the world, ranging from 0.4/100 000 for women in the state of Utah, to 170/100 000 in northern Iran. In the UK and Ireland the incidence is about 8/100 000. In the USA the incidence is higher for black males, at 12.4 per 100 000, than for white males, at 4.1 per 100 000. For black females it is 2.6 while white females have an incidence of 1 per 100 000.

The incidence is increasing along the western European seaboard, especially in England and Wales, Ireland, Scotland and Spain. This change has been accompanied by a dramatic change in the histological type. Until relatively recently, up to 95% of oesophageal cancers were squamous cell tumours. While the incidence of squamous cell lesions has remained static, the incidence of adenocarcinoma, the second most common type, has increased dramatically. In one study there was an annual average increase in oesophageal adenocarcinoma of 9.4% amongst white men and 9.8% amongst black men over a recent decade. Adenocarcinoma now accounts for 30–60% of tumours presenting to many western units. This rate of increase surpassed that of any other cancer, outpacing increases in incidence of malignant melanoma, non-Hodgkin's lymphoma and cancers of the lung.

3. The most important aetiological risk factors for squamous carcinoma are smoking, alcohol, nitrosamines, ingestion of hot liquids, mineral deficiencies, nutritional deficiencies of vitamin A, B and C and certain fungal infections. Pure ethanol is not considered to be mutagenic *per se* but appears to facilitate the diffusion of small molecules to the basal layers. Alcohol abuse, however, is usually associated with nutritional deficiency and in developing countries is occasionally contaminated by carcinogenic substances. Tobacco has a well-recognized role in the development of carcinoma, with pipe and cigar smoking being more of a risk than cigarette smoking, and the risk is directly linked with the tar content and number smoked. Exposure to nitroso compounds may occur through ingested food, water, tobacco and industrial emissions or they may be formed endogenously by the reaction of nitrites with secondary and tertiary amines. Nitrites may in turn be formed by the action of bacteria on exogenous nitrates. Pickled and stored vegetables, cured fish and meats, vegetables and alcoholic beverages are the

principal sources of nitrates. Mineral deficiencies may lead to an accumulation of nitrates and nitrites in vegetables. Plant health is compromised, predisposing to contamination by fungi. Fungal infection is known to stimulate hyperkeratosis and hyperplasia of the basal cell layer of the oesophagus.

Little is known about the risk factors for adenocarcinoma, apart from the link with Barrett's oesophagus and previous peptic ulceration or previous ulcer surgery. Barrett's in turn is due to increased incidence of gastro-oesophageal reflux. There is no clear evidence that the incidence of gastro-oesophageal reflux has increased in incidence as such studies are lacking.

4. Three randomized trials have shown no survival advantage for preoperative radiotherapy over surgery alone. A further three randomized trials have failed to demonstrate a survival advantage for postoperative radiotherapy over surgery alone. No randomized trial has yet compared preoperative chemotherapy or postoperative chemotherapy with surgery alone. Combined chemotherapy and radiotherapy preoperatively appear to confer a survival advantage for both squamous and adenocarcinoma but the trials to prove this conclusively are ongoing. No trial has properly assessed postoperative combined chemotherapy and radiotherapy for oesophageal carcinoma.

5. The prognosis for oesophageal adenocarcinoma is similar to that for squamous carcinoma. The prognosis for females, however, is significantly better than that for males, especially for premenopausal females. The reason is unclear but studies suggest a difference in behaviour of the tumour between the sexes. It is possible that the endocrine milieu in premenopausal women may prevent the establishment of micrometastases. In one large study females had earlier tumours with a lower incidence of lymph node involvement or adventitial invasion. Even tumours of similar stage were associated with significantly longer survival in the female. Lymphocytic infiltration was more frequent in the female carrying an improved prognosis.

Further reading

Blot WJ, Devesa SS, Kneller RW and Fraumeni JF. (1991) Rising incidence of adenocarcinoma of the oesophagus and gastric cardia. *Journal of the American Medical Association* **265**: 1287–1289

Cheng KK, Day NE and Davies TW. (1900) Oesophageal cancer in Europe: paradoxical time trends in relation to smoking and drinking. *British Journal of Cancer* **65**: 613–617

Hennessy TPJ and Cuschieri A. (1992) *Surgery of the Oesophagus*, 2nd edn. Butterworth-Heinemann, Oxford

Spechler SJ, Robbins AH, Rubins HB *et al.* (1984) Adenocarcinoma and Barrett's esophagus: an overrated risk? *Gastroenterology* **87**: 927–933

Thomas Noel Walsh

Case 34 Pyloric stenosis

A 4-week-old female infant was admitted for investigation of failure to thrive. She was born at 33 weeks' gestation weighing 2.2 kg with good Apgar scores and not requiring ventilation. She was discharged at 10 days of age but had lost weight since then. Her mother described her as a 'sicky baby' who vomited frequently after all feeds but who remained well in herself. The vomiting was of milk only. She had not opened her bowels for 2 days and was having fewer wet nappies than before.

Examination revealed a wasted, jaundiced baby with low-volume pulses and cool peripheries. A subsequent upper gastrointestinal contrast study showed active gastric peristalsis, delayed gastric emptying and a thin, elongated pyloric canal.

Questions

1. What is the diagnosis?
2. In what way is this baby not typical?
3. What is the differential diagnosis?
4. What biochemical disturbance is associated with this condition?
5. Describe the operation.
6. What are the potential complications?

Answers

1. The diagnosis is almost certainly that of pyloric stenosis. The features on contrast study are typical. An ultrasound examination would show hypoechoic pyloric muscle. The muscle thickness is usually greater than 4 mm and the pyloric tumour usually greater than 17 mm in length. The diagnosis could be confirmed by doing a test feed. If the baby's abdomen is palpated during the course of the feed, the pyloric tumour can usually be felt if the examiner, using the left hand, examines from the baby's left side.
2. The majority of babies with pyloric stenosis do not vomit in the first 2–3 weeks of life. The majority of babies are male, in a ratio of 4:1. Most are full-term infants and they vomit force-

fully directly after feeds.
3. Differential diagnosis would include severe gastro-oesophageal reflux and a proximal duodenal stenosis. In both cases a contrast study is required to establish or rule out the diagnosis.
4. The usual biochemical disturbance is of hypokalaemic alkalosis. This is the result of continual loss of hydrogen ion by persistent vomiting with retention of bicarbonate. In response the kidney excretes potassium while retaining hydrogen ions in order to correct the alkalosis.
5. The abdomen may be entered through a variety of incisions. Upper transverse, midline epigastric and curved supra-umbilical all have their advocates and all are appropriate. Once the pylorus is delivered, the muscle is incised longi-tudinally down to the mucosa. Using a mosquito forceps or a pyloric spreader the muscle is then widely split. At the distal end the tear in the muscle then extends obliquely and this confirms that the pyloromyotomy is adequate.
6. The commonest operative complication is of duodenal per-foration. This is usually recognized at the time and the duo-denum closed with interrupted 6/0 absorbable synthetic sutures. Perforation is the result of trying to divide the last few fibres of the pyloric tumour and this is an unnecessary manoeuvre.

   Postoperative infection is commoner after using the umbi-lical incision. Nevertheless, in these babies staphylococcal carriage in the healing umbilicus is usual. Consequently, most surgeons will use antistaphylococcal prophylaxis with induction of anaesthesia.

   Wound disruption is a particular association of pyloric stenosis. The reasons for this are not clear. My own prefer-ence for wound closure is for a mass closure technique using absorbable, synthetic sutures. Nevertheless, the reason for the higher rate of disruption in this condition has not been explained.

Further reading

Lobe TE. (1994) Pyloromyotomy. In: *Rob and Smith Operative Surgery: Paediatric Surgery* (eds Coran AG and Spitz L), 5th edn. Chapman and Hall, London

E.M. Kiely

Case 35   Oesophageal rupture

A 58-year-old woman, previously fit and healthy, awoke in the night with nausea. Shortly after, she vomited violently and returned to bed. The following morning she complained of severe, constant pain in the centre of her chest and the epigastric region. She was admitted to hospital where she was found to be peripherally vasoconstricted with a blood pressure of 90/60 mmHg and a temperature of 38.7°C. A posteroanterior chest X-ray showed a left pleural effusion and air in the mediastinum. Haematological examination of a blood film provided a white cell count of $28 \times 10^9/l$.

Questions

1. What is the likely diagnosis? What is the outcome if this condition is left untreated?
2. What further investigations should be performed?
3. How should the condition be managed prior to any surgery?
4. What surgical options are available?
5. What complications of surgery may arise?

Answers

1. The patient has undergone a spontaneous oesophageal rupture. This is known as Boerhaave's syndrome. During violent vomiting a longitudinal tear will have been created at the cardia and along the lower oesophagus with spillage of gastric contents into the mediastinum and the left pleural space. Gas tracks up beneath the mediastinal pleura and into the inferior pulmonary ligament and will eventually track out of the thoracic cavity. The finding of subcutaneous emphysema is present in most patients.

   Mediastinitis secondary to oesophageal rupture is considered to be a lethal complication if not treated expeditiously. The least morbidity and mortality is associated with prompt repair of the leak and drainage of the pleural cavity within 12 h. Here mortality may be reduced to around 10% in otherwise fit patients.

2. A Gastrografin swallow will confirm the diagnosis and localize the site of tear. Endoscopy is generally not recommended in a moribund patient where this procedure may either worsen the tear or increase the spillage of gastric contents into the chest.

3. Prompt preoperative management of oesophageal rupture will optimize the condition of the patient for surgery and maximize the chances of survival. The patient should be kept nil-by-mouth. Appropriate fluid replacement therapy should be instituted intravenously and parenteral antibiotics should be commenced immediately. The pleural effusion should be drained with a large-bore intercostal drain connected to an underwater seal bottle. Once stabilized the patient should be transferred to a specialist unit for definitive treatment of the tear.

4. It is generally recognized that delay in surgical management or even non-surgical management is associated with high mortality and for this reason expeditious surgery is recommended. With single-lung ventilation under general anaesthesia, a left thoracotomy is performed and the spilt gastric contents are aspirated from the left pleural space. Whilst performing the thoracotomy the muscles and vessels of the relevant intercostal space are preserved so that they can be separated anteriorly, left attached posteriorly, and swung down into the chest for use as a patch to repair the rupture. Direct closure and then reinforcement with such a vascularized pedicle or indeed, use of such a pedicle as a patch is associated with the best results. An alternative is the use of the fundus of the stomach.

When the edges of the oesophageal rupture are very damaged or weak or if diagnosis has been delayed, it may not be possible to perform a satisfactory repair. Under these circumstances it is possible to place a T-tube in the oesophagus to drain gastric contents outside the chest.

Finally, if rupture is found to be associated with oesophageal malignancy an oesophageal resection may be appropriate.

Following whichever procedure is chosen a nasogastric tube is left in place within the stomach and the pleural space is washed out with copious volumes of warm antiseptic solution. The chest is now closed over tap chest drains. Before leaving the operating theatre a dedicated intravenous feeding line should be sited for parenteral nutrition.

In the postoperative period it is important that antibiotics are continued. The patient should be kept nil-by-mouth and the nasogastric tube should be left on free drainage with hourly suction to minimize the chance of gastric contents washing up to the repair and exacerbating any anastomotic leak. Chest drains should be left *in situ* on free drainage. Parenteral nutrition should continue. The patient should be closely monitored for any evidence of continuing sepsis or leak with daily white cell counts and chest X-rays. A Gastrografin swallow should be performed, usually about 7 days after procedure, and if at this time no leak is demonstrated and bowel sounds have resumed the patient may be cautiously reintroduced to oral fluids and subsequently food.

5. Complications which may ensue following surgical intervention include unremitting mediastinitis and sepsis with death, the development of a fistula between the oesophagus and skin, empyema and late stricture formation within the oesophagus at the site of repair. Sepsis should be treated on its own merits with drainage and antibiotics as appropriate. Fistulas will close given adequate distal drainage into the stomach. Stricture formation can be dealt with by serial dilatation once the oesophagus is well-healed.

Further reading

Shields TW. (1994) *General Thoracic Surgery*. Section XXI Trauma to the oesophagus. Williams & Wilkins, Baltimore

Jonathan Forty

Case 36   Hazards of blood transfusion

A 69-year-old woman attended the preclerking clinic prior to admission for resection of an abdominal aortic aneurysm. She has three children from two partners and has never received a blood transfusion. She expresses concern that she may 'catch something' if she has a blood transfusion.

She is admitted 24 h later via casualty with evidence that the aneurysm has ruptured and proceeds to emergency surgery where she receives 12 units of packed red cells. She makes a satisfactory recovery, but 10 days later is noted to have a low-grade pyrexia with no evidence of infection and has become anaemic with hyperbilirubinaemia, a raised lactate dehydrogenase and positive direct antiglobulin test.

Questions

1. For which infections is donated blood routinely screened?
2. What other measures are taken to exclude alternative possible infections with blood transfusion?
3. What do you understand by the term massive blood transfusion?
4. What are the possible complications of massive blood transfusion?
5. What type of transfusion reaction has developed and how would you manage it?
6. Discuss the causes and management of the other immunologically mediated transfusion reaction.

Answers

1. Infections specifically screened are hepatitis B and hepatitis C, human immunodeficiency virus (HIV)1 and 2 and syphilis. Malaria is avoided by excluding non-immune donors who have travelled to endemic areas within the past 12 months. Cytomegalovirus (CMV) antibody is screened in a proportion to enable CMV-negative blood to be available for immunocompromised patients and neonates.

Hepatitis A is not associated with blood transfusion. Hepatitis B is a plasma-borne infection in the chronic carrier state and is excluded by testing for hepatitis B surface antigen (HBsAg). The incidence of detection is 1/11 000 donations. The diagnosis of acute hepatitis B by hepatitis B core antibody is not appropriate for donor screening to exclude carriers. Hepatitis C antibody is screened. Surrogate markers for hepatic disease, e.g. alanine aminotransferase levels, are not measured.

HIV 1 and 2 are excluded by antibody screen – HIV 1 has been screened since 1985. At-risk donors are excluded by history. A 3-month window between infection and seroconversion remains a risk period during which an infected donor could be missed. However, seroconverting donors are extremely rare, with only one instance of HIV transmission from a negative donor since screening began in 1985. Syphilis is excluded by routine screen, preferably using the *Treponema pallidum* haemagglutinin assay (TPHA) rather than the less specific Venereal Disease Research Laboratory (VDRL), which has other positive causes, e.g. Yaws.

2. Infection is excluded by the principle of using non-remunerated volunteer blood donors in whom lifestyle risks have been excluded by questionnaire, including a history of recent foreign travel to areas in which blood-borne infections are endemic.

Opportunistic infections which may complicate blood transfusion include bacterial contamination at the time of collection (staphylococci) or donor bacteraemia – a history of recent dental work is a contraindication to donation. Endotoxin-mediated damage from Gram-negative contamination is minimized by using a closed system during testing and processing. Bacterial contamination should always be suspected if the unit demonstrates haemolysis or contains clots.

In endemic areas other infections to be excluded include trypanosomiasis (Chagas disease, *Trypanosoma cruzei*), babesiosis (Nantucket fever) and human T-cell lymphotrophic virus (HTLV) 1 (acute T-cell lymphotrophic leukaemia and tropical spastic paresis).

3. Massive blood transfusion is the transfusion of a volume equal to the patient's total blood volume in less than 24 h. The aims are to maintain blood composition within limits that are safe with regard to haemostasis, blood oxygen-

carrying capacity, oncotic pressure and plasma biochemistry (British Committee for Standards in Haematology, 1988).
4. The problems of massive blood transfusion include over-/undertransfusion, thrombocytopenia, coagulation factor deficiency, impaired oxygen-carrying capacity, hypocalcaemia, hyperkalaemia and hypothermia.
Blood volume replacement may be difficult to assess accurately but other intercurrent problems are aggravated by under- or over-transfusion. Acceptable parameters as a minimum include a normal systolic blood pressure and pulse rate, urine output of 30 ml/h and a haematocrit of 0.32.
Dilutional thrombocytopenia is to be expected during massive blood transfusion. Blood which has been stored for more than a few days is devoid of functional platelets, although at least 1.5 blood volumes (7–8 l for adults) must be transfused before problems are likely. A minimal platelet count of 50×10^9/l should maintain adequate haemostasis.

Coagulation factor deficiency is not a frequent problem despite common presumptions. Stored whole blood contains adequate amounts of all coagulation factors except factor V and factor VIII, which decay during storage with levels of 5–20% at 20 days. These reduced levels are compensated for by the potent stimulus to factor VIII synthesis and release produced by the stress of trauma and surgery. Pure dilutional loss of coagulation activity is expected to be mild. Significantly disordered haemostasis is more usually due to disseminated intravascular coagulation, confirmed by thrombocytopenia $< 50 \times 10^9$/l, prolonged prothrombin time, activated partial thromboplastin time and thrombin time, a reduced fibrinogen or raised fibrinogen degradation products (FDPs). Formulaic use of fresh frozen plasma after 1 whole blood volume replacement is not indicated (British Committee for Standards in Haematology, 1992) and indiscriminate use of blood components can be avoided by early and frequent monitoring of haemostasis to direct replacement therapy.

Impaired tissue oxygenation is not a significant clinical problem despite the reduced 2,3-diphosphoglycerate (2,3-DPG) levels in stored blood, resulting in a high oxygen affinity. Clinical evidence for reduced oxygen availability to the tissues has not been forthcoming, although the use of fairly fresh blood (<1 week storage) is an acceptable compromise. 2,3-DPG regeneration is rapid after transfusion and is complete within a few hours of transfusion. Fresh whole blood is not indicated for use in massive blood transfusion as a source of coagulation factors or to enhance tissue oxygen delivery.

Hypocalcaemia is a theoretical problem as citrate used as anticoagulant binds plasma calcium, reducing plasma levels. A healthy adult liver metabolizes citrate at rates equal to 1 unit of transfused blood every 5 min. Hypocalcaemia is not a problem in healthy adults, but may be in hypothermia and in neonates with immature hepatic function.

Hyperkalaemia may result from potassium leakage from red cells, but it is not a major problem unless large amounts of blood are being given very quickly.

Hypothermia may occur and blood warmers should be used for infusion rates exceeding 1 unit/10 min in adults, time permitting.

5. The features are those of a delayed haemolytic transfusion reaction.

   Patients previously exposed to blood from transfusion or pregnancy may be immunized to foreign red cell antigens. However, the level of antibody may be at a level low enough to avoid detection on routine antibody screening during the cross-match procedure. Subsequent blood transfusion may re-expose the patient to the relevant antigen, provoking an anamnestic response.

   As a consequence, haemolysis of the transfused red cells may occur as the antibody level rises, producing a delayed haemolytic transfusion reaction. The clinical features are fever, falling haemoglobin and hyperbilirubinaemia or haemoglobinuria, typically 5–10 days after transfusion. Repeat serology may show a positive direct antiglobulin test, and the presence of an atypical antibody in the patient's serum which had been previously absent.

6. Immune-mediated transfusion reactions are:

   Immediate haemolytic transfusion reaction.
   Delayed haemolytic transfusion reaction.
   Febrile transfusion reactions.
   Transfusion-related acute lung injury.
   Transfusion-associated graft-versus-host disease (TAGvHD).
   Post-transfusion purpura.
   Urticaria.

(a) Febrile transfusion reaction. White cells may stimulate the development of antibodies to granulocyte antigens, which subsequently produce a characteristic reaction during the course of a red-cell infusion. Fever occurring 30–60 min after commencing transfusion reflects cytokine release and endogenous pyrogen formation with related shivering or rigors, but no hypotension, lumbar or chest pain. Treatment is symptomatic relief with paracetamol and slowing of the transfusion. The problem may be avoided by the use of leuko-depleted blood products, either by bedside filtration or the provision of leuko-depleted blood products from the local blood transfusion centre.

(b) Transfusion-related acute lung injury. This very rare complication of blood transfusion has been reported in 70 cases but is underdiagnosed or not recognized. Mortality is 10%. It occurs when donor plasma contains antibodies which agglutinate white cells, resulting in chills, fever, non-productive cough and dyspnoea. Chest X-ray shows numerous nodules which are predominantly perihilar and infiltration in the lower lung fields.

(c) Transfusion-associated graft-versus-host disease. This is another rare complication, probably identical with the phenomenon of postoperative erythroderma. It is 90–100% fatal. TAGvHD occurs when immunocompetent lymphocytes from the donation survive and respond in the recipient. This occurs when there is genetic similarity between donor and recipient, e.g. directed donations from family members, or when the recipient is immunocompromised. The clinical picture starts with a rash progressing to hepatitis, gastrointestinal involvement and bone marrow aplasia. No effective therapy exists, but TAGvHD can be prevented by irradiating cellular blood products prior to infusion. Irradiated products should be used for intrauterine blood transfusions, in immunocompromised hosts (congenital, acquired or iatrogenic) and also in patients with Hodgkin's disease where patients are effectively immunocompromised by their disease.

(d) Anaphylaxis. Red cell antigens and antibodies are the most important because of the relatively large volumes of red cells being transfused, the occurrence of naturally occurring complement-activating antibodies to the ABO antigens and the risk of stimulating immunoglobulin G (IgG) antibodies causing haemolytic disease of the newborn in young women.

Immediate haemolytic transfusion reactions are due to ABO incompatibility, which has a 10% mortality rate. They are not due to serological or laboratory error but are due to clerical or administrative error, including incorrect identification of the patient when taking samples, mislabelling of blood bottles and failure to comply with correct procedure when transfusing the blood.

Signs and symptoms are due to complement-mediated intravascular haemolysis after transfusion. Major ABO incompatibility is characterized by a rapid onset of symptoms following the onset of transfusion. A few millilitres of ABO-incompatible blood may cause symptoms within minutes. The clinical features include local venous pain and discomfort, headache and facial flushing, vomiting and loin pain. Symptoms include tachycardia and hypotension, rigors and pyrexia, progressing to acute renal failure with oliguria and disseminated intravascular coagulation.

The immediate management consists of stopping the transfusion, restoration of the circulation and blood volume with crystalloid and the maintenance of urinary output with intravenous frusemide 80–120 mg, given expectantly, and further renal support as required.

Recheck all available documentation and inform the laboratory immediately. Return the units of blood and send patient samples for a full blood count, repeat serology for blood grouping, direct antiglobulin test, antibody screen and compatibility testing. The suspected units should be compared with the pre- and post-transfusion serum. Further investigation should include coagulation studies, bilirubin, haptoglobins, haemoglobinaemia and haemoglobinuria, which should be monitored for 24 h. Send blood cultures from the unit to exclude bacterial contamination.

Pyrexia without any other features is unlikely to be due to red cell incompatibility, and can be managed with antipyretics and slowing of the transfusion.

(e) Post-transfusion purpura is a rare complication analogous to the delayed haemolytic reaction. A total of 1% of recipients are negative for platelet-specific antigens, usually human platelet antigen-la (HPA-la, formerly Pl^{A1}), and they may develop alloimmune antibodies, usually due to pregnancy. Blood transfusion is followed by severe thrombocytopenia 7–10 days later. Although the patient's own platelets lack the antigen, they are consumed either by cross-reaction with the antibody or as part of the immune complex formation. Although self-limiting, thrombocytopenia is severe and may result in haemorrhage. Treatment is prompt plasma exchange or intravenous immunoglobulin infusion.

(f) Urticaria and severe anaphylaxis. Mild urticarial reactions are relatively common during blood transfusion and are easily managed with antihistamines. Severe anaphylaxis with wheeze, dyspnoea and shock is very rare. It most frequently occurs in patients with IgA deficiency who have an anti-IgA antibody. Following a severe anaphylactic reaction to blood products, anti-IgA antibodies should be sought and if found, future blood products from IgA-deficient donors used. If not due to IgA antibodies, then washed cells may be used.

References and further reading

British Committee for Standards in Haematology, Working Party Blood of the Transfusion Task Force (1988) Guidelines for massive blood transfusion. *Clinical and Laboratory Haematology* **10**: 265–273

British Committee for Standards in Haematology, Working Party Blood of the Transfusion Task Force (1992) Guidelines for the use of fresh frozen plasma. *Transfusion Medicine* **2**: 57–63

British Committee for Standards in Haematology, Working Party Blood of the Transfusion Task Force (1992) Guidelines for platelet transfusions. *Transfusion Medicine* **2**: 311–318

Contreras M (ed.) (1993) *ABC of Transfusion*, 2nd edn. BMJ, London

Peter Alton

Case 37 Pancreatic cancer

A 64-year-old man consulted his general practitioner because he had felt generally unwell for a number of weeks. On direct questioning he admitted to a loss of 10 kg in body weight, dropping from about 75 to 65 kg over a 3-month period. He had lost interest in food but was drinking plenty and now had to get up twice a night to pass urine. He complained of mild discomfort in the back. Physical examination was unremarkable. The doctor found glycosuria on dipstick testing and referred him to the local diabetic physician. Two weeks later, before his out-patient appointment, the patient returned to the general practitioner's surgery because he was 'off colour', his urine was consistently dark and his stools were pale and greasy. A mass could now be felt in the right upper quadrant and there was clear-cut icterus. The doctor redirected the referral to the surgical clinic and requested an urgent appointment.

Questions

1. What is the probable diagnosis?
2. What is the explanation for the abdominal mass?
3. How should he be investigated?
4. What are the options for surgical treatment?
5. What preoperative precautions should be taken?
6. What is the prognosis?

Answers

1. Carcinoma of the head of pancreas. The non-specific pro-dromal symptoms – malaise, anorexia, weight loss – are all too common in this disease. Back pain is another typical symptom. Ultimately obstructive jaundice develops as the tumour encircles the common bile duct. Although the jaundice is of recent origin, it is likely to deepen rapidly and remorselessly, unlike the situation with gallstones, where some fluctuation is much more common. The other types of periampullary cancer – bile duct, ampulla, duodenum – will often present with obstructive jaundice, but typically this is less rapidly progressive than in pancreatic cancer.

The recent onset of diabetes mellitus is highly suggestive of carcinoma of the pancreas. It explains the polydipsia and polyuria and it probably contributed to the weight loss; other factors are the tumour itself and the exocrine pancreatic insufficiency that often follows neoplastic obstruction of the pancreatic duct (note the hint of steatorrhoea). The explanation for glucose intolerance in pancreatic cancer is uncertain. It is not just a matter of neoplastic replacement of the islet cell tissue, but may possibly involve the secretion of an anti-insulin. Pancreatic cancer is probably commoner in diabetics than the general population, and in such circumstances it may be heralded by an increased insulin requirement.

2. The abdominal mass probably represents a distended gallbladder. Neither the primary tumour nor any hepatic secondaries are likely to have become palpable over a 2-week period, though the development of obstructive jaundice might have led the general practitioner to examine the abdomen more thoroughly on the second occasion. Courvoisier's law dictates that the presence of a mass in a jaundiced patient makes the diagnosis one of cancer and not gallstones. Thus a palpable gallbladder is a most useful physical sign. I do not believe one suggested explanation for Courvoisier's law, namely that a gallbladder that produces stones is incapable of distension, since I have encountered several patients with concomitant gallstones and pancreatic cancer in whom the organ was clearly palpable. To my mind the explanation for Courvoisier's law is that neoplastic obstruction of the bile duct is much more complete than gallstone obstruction, in which the calculus acts as a ball valve and permits partial decompression of the biliary tree.

3. Investigation starts with a full blood count and liver function tests, which should be repeated to show the typical rise in serum bilirubin and alkaline phosphatase; elevations in transaminases are modest unless cholangitis supervenes. An ultrasound scan of the right upper quadrant will reveal dilatation of the gallbladder and of the intra- and extrahepatic biliary tree. It helps to rule out gallstones and 'medical' causes of jaundice such as hepatitis and drugs. Ultrasound may demonstrate a pancreatic mass and secondary spread (hepatic metastases, ascites). Computed tomography (CT) scan supplements this information in a format that can readily be appreciated by the clinician. In my experience CT

scan is superior to ultrasound in demonstrating the primary tumour and its crucial relationship to the portal vein (see below), but it may not give precise information about tumour size. Magnetic resonance imaging does not yet provide superior imaging, but the situation may change as the technology improves.

Endoscopic retrograde cholangiopancreatography (ERCP) is an important investigation, demonstrating the level and the nature of the bile duct stricture and concomitant involvement of the pancreatic duct (the 'double duct' sign). Brushings of the stricture or scrutiny of the pancreatic juice will sometimes provide cytological confirmation of cancer. Ampullary and duodenal cancers can be directly seen and biopsied. If ERCP fails, percutaneous transhepatic cholangiography (PTC) produces much of the same information. I do not bother with percutaneous biopsy of a pancreatic mass if I plan to resect it, but I do obtain visceral angiography to show any major arterial or venous encasement and to demonstrate the arterial anomalies that are frequently present in the general population. Laparoscopy and laparoscopic ultrasound may also have a role in staging pancreatic cancer and ruling out needless laparotomy.

4. In my judgement a *resectable* tumour of the pancreas should be resected. A tumour may be irresectable because of patient factors (age, frailty, intercurrent disease) or tumour factors (hepatic or peritoneal metastases, portal vein invasion). Resection involves pancreatoduodenectomy, and the pylorus-preserving modification may be appropriate if the tumour does not lie close to the duodenal cap. The operative mortality rate should not exceed 10% if resection is to be an appropriate option. Total pancreatectomy and regional lymphadenectomy have a very limited role; adjuvant oncological treatment is of uncertain value.

If the tumour is clearly irresectable on imaging and a short survival is anticipated, the bile duct stricture should be stented by either the endoscopic or the percutaneous route; expandable metal stents last longer than plastic (polythene) tubes. If there is any doubt about the diagnosis or the resectability of the tumour and the patient does not belong to a high-risk category, I have little hesitation in adopting a surgical approach to palliation. Laparotomy allows a clear-cut diagnosis to be reached with accurate staging of the tumour. Jaundice is corrected by means of choledochojejunostomy Roux-en-Y; the gallbladder is a poor conduit because of subsequent tumour encroachment on the cystic duct. Vomiting is prevented by synchronous gastroenterostomy, and pain can be relieved by intraoperative blockade of the coeliac plexus using 50% alcohol. As with resection, palliative surgery is only acceptable if the complication rate is low.

5. Any jaundiced patient represents an increased surgical risk. Dehydration is common, and preoperative intravenous infusion is often advisable to prevent the hepatorenal syndrome (postoperative renal failure). Hypoprothombinaemia is generally correctable with parenteral administration of vitamin K. The operation should be 'covered' with broad-spectrum antibiotics (e.g. gentamicin and a cephalosporin) and some form of thromboprophylaxis (e.g. subcutaneous heparin). The value of preoperative biliary decompression is unproven. Although deeply jaundiced patients are catabolic and withstand surgical complications poorly, the techniques of percutaneous and endoscopic drainage carry their own risks, notably the introduction of infection into a previously sterile biliary tree. In practice, preoperative decompression (ideally from below, i.e. at ERCP) is probably advisable for those with a serum bilirubin above 200 μmol/l for more than 1–2 weeks, and it should be undertaken as an emergency in the presence of cholangitis or severe renal insufficiency. The biliary stent is removed at the subsequent operation.

6. In general the prognosis of pancreatic cancer remains very poor. At best, only 5–10% of those who survive a 'curative' resection will be alive 5 years later, presumably because micrometastases are already present at the time of operation. In this particular patient there are certain indicators to suggest an unfavourable prognosis. Back pain is a sinister symptom, suggesting posterior extracapsular invasion. The 3-month prodromal history before the onset of jaundice suggests that the tumour may have arisen in the neck of pancreas or the uncinate process and already have spread beyond the possibility of surgical cure before causing jaundice. If the CT scan shows hepatic metastases or the angiogram shows portal vein occlusion with a collateral circulation, the tumour is incurable. It is then necessary to clinch the diagnosis by percutaneous biopsy of the primary or secondary tumour and to relieve the jaundice by a biliary stent (see above). Thereafter it is my practice to obtain an

oncological opinion since radiotherapy and/or chemotherapy can probably prolong life in individual cases even if no clear statistical benefit has been shown in prospective trials. One final point is worth mentioning: no patient should be told that he or she definitely has cancer without a positive tissue diagnosis. To forget this rule is to risk the embarrassment and potential lawsuit of the occasional erroneous diagnosis, since chronic pancreatitis can closely mimic pancreatic cancer.

Further reading

Watanapa P and Williamson RCN. (1992) Surgical palliation for pancreatic cancer: developments during the last two decades. *British Journal of Surgery* **79**: 8–20

Watanapa P and Williamson RCN. (1995) Resection of the pancreatic head with or without gastrectomy. *World Journal of Surgery* **19**: 403–409

R.C.N. Williamson

Case 38   Phaeochromocytoma

A 51-year-old female accountant presented to her general practitioner with an 18-month history of 'funny turns' which tended
to occur in the morning when she felt hot and developed palpitations, nausea and vomiting. These attacks were often associated with severe headache. Physical examination was
unremarkable. The full blood count and biochemical profile
were normal, and the erythrocyte sedimentation rate was
56 mm/h. When the patient reattended the doctor's surgery for
these results, she suffered a further attack. The doctor wit-
nessed that the patient was very pale and recorded the blood
pressure at 220/110 mmHg. The doctor arranged for 24 h urine
vanillylmandelic acid (VMA) measurements which were elevated, and an urgent endocrine referral was sought.

Questions

1. What is the likely diagnosis and how would you set out to
   confirm it?
2. What other endocrine conditions are associated with phaeochromocytoma and how would you screen for them?
3. Once the diagnosis of phaeochromocytoma had been confirmed, how would you attempt to localize the tumour?
4. What steps would you take to prepare the patient before
   surgery?
5. What are the surgical approaches to resecting a phaeochromocytoma?

Answers

1. The diagnosis of a phaeochromocytoma should be considered. This is a catecholamine-secreting tumour of
   chromaffin cells which have migrated from the neural crest
   to rest either within the adrenal medulla or in the para-
   ganglionic tissues adjacent to the sympathetic chain. These
   tumours typically secrete noradrenaline, or occasionally
   adrenaline and, rarely, dopamine and a variety of other

neurotransmitters, in an episodic manner. Excessive alpha-adrenoceptor stimulation leads to vasoconstriction and a reduced intravascular volume and beta-1 receptors may respond to this effect with a reflex tachycardia. Phaeochromocytomas become clinically manifest by episodic headaches, palpitations and excessive sweating associated with systemic hypertension.

Clinical examination is often normal, but may reveal an abdominal tumour, hypertension or postural hypotension. The haematocrit may be raised secondary to a reduced circulatory volume and electrocardiography may reveal cardiac hypertrophy secondary to sustained hypertension. Twenty-four-hour urinary VMA measurement is an effective screening test for phaeochromocytoma. VMA, a common metabolite of noradrenaline and adrenaline, is excreted into the urine and the patient is required to adhere to a strict exclusion diet before and during the urine collection period. If the 24-h measurement is elevated, a number of special investigations are available to confirm the diagnosis:

(a) Urine measurements of either noradrenaline/adrenaline or their metabolites normetanephrine/metanephrine will be elevated in phaeochromocytoma.

(b) The gold-standard test is measurement of plasma concentrations of noradrenaline and adrenaline.

(c) When the results of the above tests are borderline, two suppression tests are available to prove or exclude phaeochromocytoma in patients with hypertension. Clonidine (alpha-2 receptor agonist) and pentolinium (inhibitor of noradrenaline or adrenaline release by sympathetic overactivity) suppress catecholamine concentrations in patients without a phaeochromocytoma.

2. Phaeochromocytoma occurs in approximately half of patients with the multiple endocrine neoplasia (MEN) type II syndrome; however, the distribution of the tumour is different – they are bilateral in up to 70% of cases and extra-adrenal tumours and malignant changes are rare. The hallmark tumour in MEN II is medullary carcinoma of the thyroid, a neoplasm derived from the C cells of the thyroid. These tumours secrete calcitonin, and can therefore be screened by measuring the basal plasma calcitonin concentration, and again following stimulation with intravenous pentagastrin (pentagastrin stimulation test). Parathyroid hyperplasia leading to primary hyperparathyroidism is the

third endocrine anomaly in the MEN II syndrome. Patients are screened by measuring plasma calcium concentration, followed by parathyroid hormone assay if the plasma calcium is elevated. Recent research has identified a genetic marker in the DNA of affected patients. The RET proto-oncogene encodes a tyrosine kinase receptor and suggests that the underlying defect is a loss of control in the proliferation of neural crest cells. This RET proto-oncogene has been detected in patients with sporadic medullary carcinoma of the thyroid, MEN II (a, b) and Hirschsprung's disease, whose common link is a disorder of cells derived from the neural crest.

Phaeochromocytoma is also associated with various neuroectodermal disorders including von Hippel–Lindau disease (phaeochromocytoma, angioma, renal carcinoma), neurofibromatosis (1 % of cases) and tuberous sclerosis.

3. Localization of the tumour should not be attempted until the diagnosis has been confirmed biochemically as non-functioning adrenal adenomas and benign extra-adrenal tumours are not uncommon, and are becoming increasingly recognized as greater numbers of patients are subjected to abdominal ultrasound and computed tomographic (CT) scanning.

Phaeochromocytomas are known as the '10% tumour' because 10% are bilateral, 10% lie outside the adrenal gland in any place where nests of primitive neural crest cells have survived, extending from the base of the skull to the epididymis, and 10% are malignant (2–11% intra-adrenal vs 30–40% in extra-adrenal tumours).

The ideal initial localization procedure would be a ^{131}I-meta-iodo-benzyl guanidine (MIBG) scan. MIBG is an analogue of noradrenaline and guanethidine which is actively concentrated in chromaffin cells. An MIBG scan is a non-invasive whole-body scan and is particularly beneficial in extra-adrenal, multiple and metastatic tumours. Its findings should be supported by other imaging modalities (CT, ultrasound). MIBG is taken up by the thyroid and patients should therefore be blocked with Lugol's iodine prior to scanning.

CT scanning provides excellent images of the adrenals. Urographic contrast can precipitate hypertensive crises and patients should already be controlled on alpha-blockade. Magnetic resonance imaging (MRI) scanning provides equal-quality images of the adrenals compared with CT but has distinct resolution advantages over extra-adrenal sites. MRI incurs no radiation exposure and is therefore the modality of choice in pregnancy.

In circumstances where the above techniques have failed to localize the tumour (no adrenal mass on CT and negative MIBG), selective venous sampling may be considered. This invasive test involves percutaneous venous catheterization and measuring plasma noradrenaline/adrenaline concentrations at various anatomical sites. Again, patients should be controlled on alpha-blockade as the procedure can provoke hypertensive crises.

4. The importance of optimal pharmacological control of the patient preoperatively is paramount. In the presence of a functional but unrecognized phaeochromocytoma, the operative mortality exceeds 50%, but this falls to less than 3% when the patient has been appropriately prepared.

   The initial step is to alpha-blockade the patient, preferably as a hospital inpatient. Phenoxybenzamine, a non-selective alpha-blocker, is the agent of choice, commencing with a dose of 5 mg/day and gradually increasing until the blood pressure is controlled. The blood volume is restored by increasing oral intake, but the patient may also require intravenous fluid transfusion. Increased blood volume can be assessed from daily weights and the haematocrit. If the patient develops a reflex tachycardia (beta stimulation secondary to alpha$_2$-blockade), then additional beta-blockade may be prescribed. Some patients may have developed myocardial damage secondary to long-term hypertension and echocardiography may be indicated. For those patients undergoing bilateral adrenalectomy, steroid replacement therapy should be commenced from the day of surgery.

5. Seven approaches to resecting a phaeochromocytoma have been described:
   (a) An anterior transperitoneal approach can be achieved via a variety of incisions (Kocher, gable, vertical and transverse). It permits access to both adrenal glands and para-aortic ganglia and allows assessment of the liver and other viscera. For these reasons it is regarded as the gold-standard approach.
   (b) Small adrenal tumours (maximal diameter less than 5 cm) may be accessed via a posterior approach. A hockey-stick incision and resection of the 12th rib provides direct access to the adrenal gland. Advantages to

this approach include less postoperative pain and avoidance of a paralytic ileus, thus shortening hospital stay. However, it is a unilateral approach and the operative field is comparatively restricted. In occasional circumstances, when the pleural cavity is entered, the pleural defect is primarily repaired with the lung fully inflated and a chest drain may be placed.

(c) The lateral loin approach under the 12th rib is popular in urology, but may result in poor access to the upper pole of the adrenal gland, particularly on the right side.

(d) In the presence of large adrenal tumours (maximum diameter greater than 15 cm) and particularly in the presence of local invasion, a thoracoabdominal approach through the 10th (right) or 11th (left) rib space provides excellent exposure to the adrenal gland and adjacent structures. If necessary, the wound can be extended into the peritoneal cavity.

(e) In the past, adrenal tumours were occasionally excised via a purely thoracic (transdiaphragmatic) approach. This technique has fallen out of favour.

(f) In rare circumstances, when a phaeochromocytoma locally invades into the renal vein and inferior vena cava, it is advantageous to gain control of the intrapericardial inferior vena cava. This can be achieved with a midline sternal division combined with a Kocher incision to access the adrenal gland – the sternocostal approach.

(g) Adrenalectomies have now been successfully performed laparoscopically, either transperitoneally or within the retroperitoneal space. Early results suggest a speedy postoperative recovery, and the only hindrance to this approach appears to be the size of the tumour.

The sequence of questions to the above case history outlines the principles of endocrine surgery:

1. Confirm the endocrine diagnosis.
2. Localize the tumour/tumours.
3. Render the patient safe.
4. Consider whether the patient needs surgery.
5. Consider the most appropriate type of operation.

Further reading

Deans GT, Kappadia R, Wedgewood K, Royston CMS and Brough WA. (1995) Laparoscopic adrenalectomy. *British Journal of Surgery* **82:** 994–995

Lynn JA and Bloom SR. (eds) (1993) *Surgical Endocrinology.* Butterworth-Heinemann, London

van Heyningen V. (1994) One gene – four syndromes. *Nature* **367:** 319–320

David M. Scott-Coombes

John A. Lynn

Case 39 Penetrating chest wound

A 28-year-old man was admitted to casualty following multiple stabbings 20 min previously. There were entry wounds in the anterior chest wall to the left of the sternum, in the lateral left chest wall, and a further two superficial wounds in the epigastric region. The weapon was a 15-cm-long knife. On admission he was conscious, tachycardic (pulse 120 beats/min), cold and sweaty, with blood pressure of 100/80 mmHg and with reduced breath sounds and dullness to percussion in the left lower zone of his chest. The ECG was normal. Chest radiography demonstrated a left haemopneumothorax only. On insertion of a left intercostal drain, 1 l of blood was evacuated together with air, followed almost immediately by progressive hypotension and bradycardia.

Questions

1. What is the diagnosis?
2. What is the mechanism for the hypotension and the delay in presentation?
3. What investigations, if any, should be undertaken?
4. What is the management of choice?
5. Is bypass essential for the management of this patient?
6. What are the possible complications on intracardiac trauma?
7. What is the postoperative management of these patients?

Answers

1. In any patient with penetrating wounds in the area of the heart, an intracardiac injury must always be suspected. This suspicion is greatly enhanced in the context of hypotension in the presence of volume replacement. Usually signs elicited from a haemodynamically compromised patient with such injuries are not useful in establishing a diagnosis unequivocally. These patients are usually too sick to detect subtle clinical signs such as Beck's triad – small quiet heart, elevated venous pressure and hypotension. A diagnosis of intrapericardial injury with tamponade, therefore, should be made.

2. The decreased cardiac output and hypotension is a result of massive blood loss, tamponade or both. The predominance of one or other is dependent on the integrity of the pericardium, which is usually good with penetrating knife wounds. Exsanguination constitutes only about 9% of stab wounds to the heart and, thus, in the majority of cases the hypotension is a result of tamponade.

   Acute tamponade is the result of a rapid increase in intrapericardial fluid with the intrapericardial pressure rising to 20–30 mmHg. In response to such a rise in pressure there is reflex vasoconstriction, catecholamine release and sodium and water retention. Thus the cardiac output is maintained by an elevation of the venous pressure. There is however a limit to this compensatory mechanism and the cardiac output will eventually fall in the presence of a persistent and rising intrapericardial pressure.

   The delay in significant haemodynamic deterioration, particularly in the young and fit, is due to the compensatory mechanisms described above. Their protective effect, however, collapses once their limit is reached, and the subsequent fall in cardiac output is progressive and fatal unless reversed.

3. Usually with intrapericardial injuries other injuries sustained can, at least in the immediate short term, be overlooked or undertreated until the dramatic intrapericardial injury is treated. In the case of this patient, further investigation is not indicated and transfer for immediate operation is mandatory. Some time may, however, be bought by a therapeutic intervention that is partly diagnostic. Pericardocentesis using a plastic intravenous catheter to enter the pericardial space via a subxiphoid approach will release enough blood (40–50 ml), and therefore enough intrapericardial pressure, to re-establish the haemodynamic situation. In diagnostic terms, however, pericardocentesis has been associated with a high incidence of false positives and negatives. Others have advocated a more formal approach by fashioning a subxiphoid pericardial window under local or light general anaesthesia in the operating room. This, however, is usually time-consuming (10–20 min in skilled hands) and adds nothing as most patients will require a subsequent midline sternotomy.

   In more stable patients with a greater degree of uncertainty regarding intrapericardial injury, further investigations may be helpful. This, however, should be undertaken only in the presence of an understanding that surgical exploration will be performed if there is a rapid deterioration in the patient's haemodynamic condition. Of the investigations available, two-dimensional echocardiography is the most useful as it will describe cardiac wall motion and cardiac valve function and detect the presence of excessive pericardial fluid. The role of cardiac catheterization for coronary angiography is doubtful unless the clinical condition is one of chronic low-grade haemodynamic compromise in the presence of new heart murmurs or ECG changes.

4. The management of choice is intrapericardial exploration. This is best performed by midline sternotomy as it provides better exposure of the great vessels, enables standard establishment of cardiopulmonary bypass if necessary and affords superior postoperative ventilatory mechanics. In this particular patient the left pleura could also be opened via the midline sternotomy and the source of left-sided chest bleeding, if present, be identified. In institutions where midline sternotomy is uncommon, anterolateral thoracotomy on the side of greatest bleeding is an alternative, with extension across the sternum if pericardial trauma is confirmed.

Bleeding should initially be controlled with digital pressure. Ventricular wounds are repaired with pledgeted sutures (Teflon or pericardium), 2-0 or 3-0 interrupted polypropylene sutures. Atrial or caval wounds are controlled usually by side-biting vascular clamps and repaired with continuous 3-0 or 4-0 polypropylene sutures. If haemorrhage is excessive, some control can be obtained by inflow occlusion of one or both cavae. If the damage is more extensive then cardiac surgical expertise should be sought. If there is widespread damage to the ventricular wall or proximal coronary arterial damage, then full heparinization and cardiopulmonary bypass may be indicated. The introduction of full heparinization should be undertaken in the knowledge of the presence of potential sites of bleeding elsewhere in the body.

5. In most cases of intrapericardial wound injury by knife, cardiopulmonary bypass is not required. It was reported necessary in 2/50 and 3/200 cases in two recently reported series. Thus, delaying management by transferring patients to hospitals with cardiopulmonary bypass facilities is contraindicated. Clearly, however, patients who have sustained

intrapericardial injuries are better managed in institutions where such facilities are available and where personnel experienced in cardiac surgery are present.

6. Stab wounds most commonly cause damage to the heart walls. With stab wounds to the front of the chest, right ventricular damage is most frequent (42%), followed by left ventricular damage. Coronary arteries are less frequently damaged and if minor or distal can be ligated. More major vessels should be repaired or, if this is not possible, grafted. Valvular and traumatic septal defects are rare and usually better tolerated by the patient and therefore managed subacutely. The defect should be repaired preserving normal tissue where possible.

7. The patient should be managed as after bypass or, if this was not instituted, as a patient who is admitted for myocardial infarction. There should be continuous monitoring for at least 24 h, particularly to detect potentially fatal dysrhythmias. Sequential ECGs and cardiac enzymes should be monitored. Any ventricular ectopic should be treated aggressively with antiarrhythmics and, if the haemodynamic situation necessitates it, a Swan–Ganz catheter should be inserted to guide inotrope manipulation. Finally, if indicated, an intra-aortic balloon pump may be used.

Further reading

Swanson J and Trunkey DD. (1989) *Trauma to the Chest Wall, Pleura and Thoracic Viscera*. In: Shields TW (ed.) *General Thoracic Surgery*, 3rd edn. pp. 465–469. Lea & Febiger, Philadelphia

Chandana Ratnatunga

Index

Page numbers in **bold** type refer to Figures or Tables